D1395192

BROKE VEGAN

OVER 100 PLANT-BASED RECIPES THAT DON'T COST THE EARTH

SASKIA SIDEY

hamlyn

First published in Great Britain in 2020 by Hamlyn,
an imprint of Octopus Publishing Group Ltd
Carmelite House
50 Victoria Embankment
London EC4Y 0DZ
www.octopusbooks.co.uk

An Hachette UK Company
www.hachette.co.uk

Photography copyright © Octopus Publishing Group 2020
Text copyright © Octopus Publishing Group 2020
Design and layout copyright © Octopus Publishing Group 2020

Distributed in the US by Hachette Book Group
1290 Avenue of the Americas
4th and 5th Floors
New York, NY 10104

Distributed in Canada by Canadian Manda Group
664 Annette St.
Toronto, Ontario
Canada M6S 2C8

ISBN 978 0 60063 698 4

A CIP catalogue record for this book is available
from the British Library.

Printed and bound in Europe

3 5 7 9 10 8 6 4 2

Commissioned by George Brooker
Copy Editor: Lucy Bannell
Senior Designer: Jaz Bahra
Photographer and Props Stylist: Jo Sidey
Food Stylist: Saskia Sidey
Production Manager: Lisa Pinnell

Standard level spoon measurements are used in all recipes.
1 tablespoon = one 15 ml spoon
1 teaspoon = one 5 ml spoon

Imperial and metric measurements have been given in all recipes.
Use one set of measurements only and not a mixture of both.

CONTENTS

SAVING THE WORLD DOESN'T NEED TO COST YOU THE EARTH

This book doesn't use any of the expensive ingredients traditionally associated with veganism. There are no 'meat alternatives' in sight. No tofu, tempeh or seitan. There is such a wide variety of fresh fruit and vegetables available that it's just not necessary for your food to pretend to be something it's not. Vegan food lends itself to saving you money as you're mainly buying fresh produce, not spending lots on expensive luxuries such as meat and dairy.

Where possible, as well as saving you money, this book aims to save you time, but there are some instances where putting in an extra few minutes at the stove will help to coax rich flavour from your ingredients, and that is worth its weight in gold. Here are some tips about how to be a Broke Vegan, so you can save money and eat better.

USE YOUR FREEZER

A freezer can help you to reduce food waste and save money. Always be on the lookout for bargain deals at your local supermarket or greengrocer and freeze any fruit or vegetables that look like they're about to be past their best for future use. Try freezing herbs in ice cube trays covered in oil. As a general rule for fruit and vegetables, only freeze things that you are going to cook once defrosted, as they won't taste as good 'raw'. Keep your freezer loaded with peas, leftover mashed potato, spinach blocks and batch-cooked meals and you'll never go hungry.

SHOP SMART

Shopping seasonally is one of the best ways to cut costs, and your fruit and vegetables will taste so much better. Out-of-season produce is often flown over internationally and the prices usually reflect that. Watch out for bargain deals and reduced items and shop towards the end of the day, when shops often slash their prices; you may need to be flexible and think on your feet, but if you can get inspired by what's on offer then you'll save a lot of cash. Buy own-brand where possible in big supermarkets, because it often works out cheaper for canned goods and pantry staples. Shop in speciality shops, such as Asian supermarkets, as well as in neighbourhood stores – you can often get up to five times the amount of dried pulses, grains and spices for the same price as their supermarket counterparts. Many supermarkets and greengrocers also sell bags of 'wonky' or 'misshapen' fruit and vegetables at a fraction of the cost of their more picture-perfect cousins.

PLAN, PLAN, PLAN

It sounds obvious but having a plan and sticking to it will help you not to waste any food and therefore save you money.

Try and stick to a meal plan for the week, cook in batches and freeze what you don't need, or aim to incorporate leftovers in your weekly menu. Try and arrange your meals around key ingredients: if some of your recipes use just a couple of sweet potatoes but you know that you can get a good deal on a big bag of them, try and incorporate more recipes into your meal plan that use them, to make sure nothing goes to waste. Only buy what you need and stick to your shopping list.

DIY

Where possible, making your own versions of shop-bought classics will save you money. Check out the recipes for Cheat's Sourdough (see page 10), multiple varieties of pesto (see pages 70–1), Any Can Hummus (see page 115) and DIY Baked Beans (see page 36) for inspiration and think about ways to cook other ready-made favourites at home.

JAZZ UP THE BASICS

Lemon or lime zest and juice, proper seasoning and a drizzle of good-quality olive oil are all instant and cheap ways to elevate your cooking. Broke food doesn't have to be bland, especially if you invest in the key ingredients outlined in Pantry Staples (see page 6).

GROW YOUR OWN

You're not expected to have a whole garden full of fruit and vegetables, but it's a great idea to invest in living herb pots from a supermarket. These are typically only fractionally more expensive than a packet of precut herbs. You only pay once and they keep replenishing themselves every time you pick some. Go for pots of basil, parsley, mint, thyme and chives on your windowsill and you'll be able to add heaps of flavour to all your dishes for years to come. Basil, coriander and parsley are also easy to grow from packets of seed, which works out even cheaper: plant them in recycled yogurt pots punctured with a few holes in the base for drainage. Or try regrowing lettuces and spring onions by submerging the rooted base in water.

PANTRY STAPLES

ESSENTIAL DRY STORES

In order to make the most of the cheapest ingredients, there are certain storecupboard staples worth investing in. Although some of them may seem expensive when you first buy them, they'll last for months and add buckets of flavour to all your dishes.

PANTRY FLAVOUR-BOMBS

Capers
Chilli oil / chilli sauce
Dijon mustard
Green olives
Harissa
Maple syrup
Yeast extract (such as Marmite)
Miso paste
Nutritional yeast
Tahini
Vanilla extract
Vegan bouillon powder

FATS & VINEGARS

You don't need every oil and vinegar on this list; most are interchangeable. If you only choose a few, go for extra virgin olive oil, sunflower oil and white wine vinegar. Sherry vinegar can be economical if you go for own-brand varieties and there are also bargains to be found if you buy extra virgin olive oil in bulk – rectangular cans are good to look out for – and pick the best-priced on the shelves.

Coconut oil
Extra virgin olive oil
Flavourless oil, such as vegetable or sunflower
Light olive oil
Vegan margarine
Apple cider vinegar
Balsamic vinegar
Sherry vinegar or red wine vinegar
White wine vinegar

DRIED HERBS & SPICES

Start with the basics, then add extras as and when you need them.

Black peppercorns
Cayenne pepper
Chilli flakes
Curry powder
Dried oregano
Fine sea salt

Ground cinnamon
Ground coriander
Ground cumin
Ground turmeric
Paprika
Whole nutmeg

EMBRACE CANS

Canned pulses, vegetables and fruit are
often not seen as fashionable, but you'll
often find the price is much lower than
their fresh equivalents.

Sweetcorn
Black beans
Butter beans
Cannellini beans or other white beans
Chickpeas
Chopped tomatoes
Kidney beans
Whole plum tomatoes

GRAINS & CARBS

Basmati rice
Couscous
Dried pasta
Rolled oats

FRESH PRODUCE
TO HAVE AROUND

Dairy-free milk, such as soy or almond
    milk
Ginger
Garlic
Lemons
Limes
Onions
Potatoes
Red chillies
Red onions
Shallots

BAKING

These staples will last for ages in your
cupboard, so stock up when you can
afford them.

Baking powder
Bicarbonate of soda
Cashew nuts
Caster sugar
Cornflour
Fast-action dried yeast
Flaked almonds
Golden syrup or light corn syrup
Ground almonds
Light brown sugar
Plain flour
Self-raising flour
Strong white bread flour

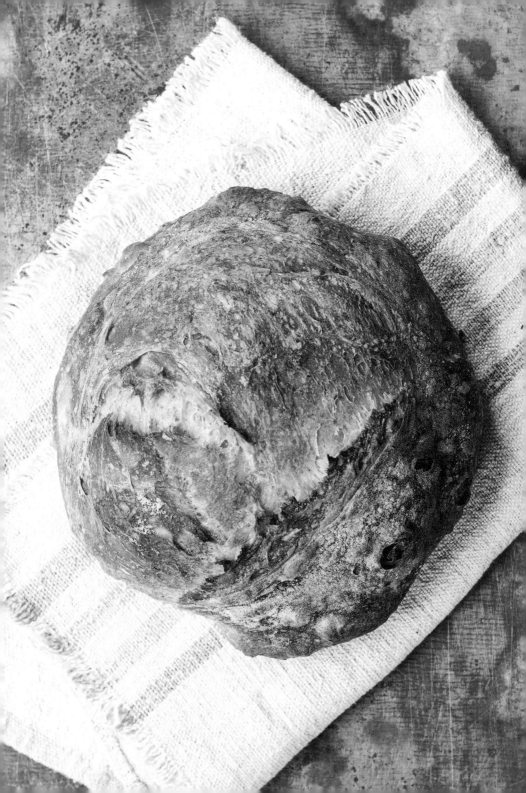

BREAKFAST & BRUNCH

CHEAT'S SOURDOUGH

The secret to this recipe is adding vinegar to lend a sour note and a slow overnight rise – you don't even have to worry about keeping a starter alive! (See photo on page 8.)

MAKES 1 LARGE LOAF

450 g (14½ oz) strong white bread flour, plus extra for dusting

50 g (2 oz) strong wholemeal bread flour

10 g (2 teaspoons) fine sea salt

scant ⅛ teaspoon fast-action dried yeast

1 teaspoon white wine vinegar

375 ml (13 fl oz) cold water

Put the flours, salt, yeast, vinegar and measured water in a large bowl and mix well until fully combined. Cover with a damp tea towel and leave at room temperature to prove overnight (12 hours).

The next morning, the dough should have risen and be bubbly. Preheat the oven as high as it can go (240°C/475°F, Gas Mark 9) and place a large cast-iron casserole dish in the oven to preheat for at least 1 hour.

Meanwhile, lightly dust a work top with flour. Wet your hands and scrape out the dough from the bowl. On the work top, fold the 4 corners of the dough inwards to the centre, then flip the dough over. Using both hands, cup the dough and pull it in a clockwise motion to create tension on the surface and help form it into a round shape. It is a very wet dough, so don't worry if you don't get the hang of it at first as it will still bake beautifully. Once you're satisfied that you have a smooth top, leave the dough uncovered for 30 minutes to rest.

After 30 minutes, lightly flour the surface of the dough and the work top and flip the dough over. Pull out the corners to make a rough square, then fold the left third of the dough into the middle, then the right third on top of that. Roll the dough up tightly, and place seam side down on a large piece of nonstick baking paper – the surface should be smooth on top. Use a sharp knife to score the top.

Lower the loaf on its paper into the casserole dish, cover and bake for 30 minutes, then remove the lid and bake for a further 20 minutes until deep golden and hollow sounding when tapped on the base. Place the loaf on a wire rack to cool. Leave for 1 hour before slicing.

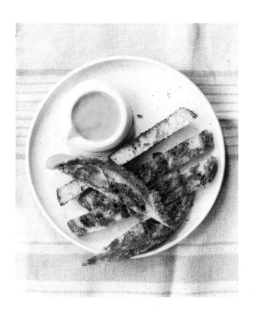

DIP WITH SOLDIERS

SERVES 2

Dip
235 ml (7½ fl oz) water
1 tablespoon cornflour
3 tablespoons nutritional
    yeast
½ teaspoon ground turmeric
salt and pepper

Toast
4 thick slices of Cheat's
    Sourdough (see opposite)
vegan margarine, for
    spreading
yeast extract (such as
    Marmite), for spreading

This salty, savoury vibrant yellow sauce is reminiscent of a dippy (soft-boiled) egg. It contains only four ingredients, is super simple to make and is the perfect vehicle for eating too much toast.

Put all the ingredients for the dip into a small saucepan. Bring to the boil over a medium heat, whisking constantly, until thickened and glossy. Season to taste.

Toast the sourdough, spread it generously with both vegan margarine and yeast extract, then slice into vertical strips to make soldiers.

Serve the sauce in egg cups or small bowls, using the soldiers to dip in.

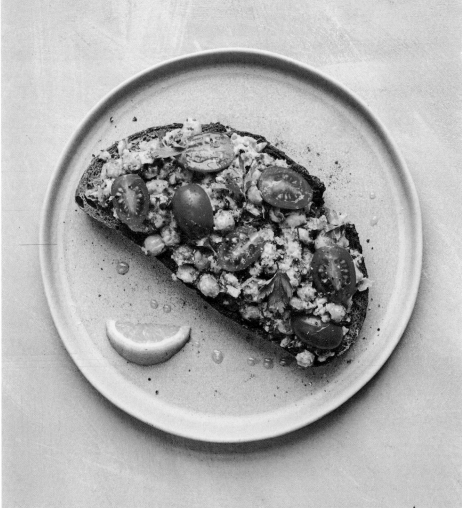

SMASHED CHICKPEAS WITH TOMATOES

If the only things you smash are avocados, you're going to rack up quite a hefty bill. Chickpeas are affordable and are amazing on toast because they take on whatever flavour you add. Try tossing them with chilli sauce or pesto for another variation.

SERVES 2

400 g (13 oz) can chickpeas, drained and rinsed

4 tablespoons tahini

2 tablespoons olive oil, plus extra for drizzling

large handful of flat leaf parsley, finely chopped, plus extra to serve

4 thick slices of Cheat's Sourdough (see page 10)

10 cherry tomatoes, halved

salt and pepper

To serve
lemon wedges
1 teaspoon paprika

Put the chickpeas in a bowl and use a potato masher to crush them, then add the tahini and olive oil and continue to crush until you reach your desired consistency. Some brands of canned chickpeas may need to be flashed in the microwave for 10–20 seconds to soften, if they prove too hard to mash.

Season with salt and pepper and fold in the parsley. Toast the bread.

Heap the chickpea mixture on the toast and top with the tomatoes. Serve with lemon wedges, a sprinkling of paprika and parsley.

BANANA FRENCH TOAST

SERVES 2

French toast is best made with stale sourdough. If the bread is really dry, splash it with a few drops of water before cooking.

1 ripe banana, plus a few extra banana slices, to serve

200 ml (7 fl oz) dairy-free milk

¼ teaspoon ground cinnamon

4 thick slices of Cheat's Sourdough (see page 10)

2 tablespoons coconut oil or vegan margarine

maple syrup, to serve

Mash the banana in a wide, shallow bowl with the back of a fork until smooth. Stir in the dairy-free milk and cinnamon.

Dip the sourdough slices in the banana milk and leave to soak while you preheat a large frying pan over a medium-high heat.

Melt 1 tablespoon of the coconut oil or margarine in the pan. Pick 2 slices of bread out of the banana milk and allow the excess to drip off, then add to the pan. Cook for 2 minutes on each side until golden and puffy, then transfer to a serving plate. Repeat with the remaining bread.

Serve with maple syrup and more banana slices.

MUSTARD & AVOCADO TOAST

SERVES 1

A combination that sounds like it shouldn't work, but does.

1 tablespoon Dijon mustard

1 tablespoon vegan mayonnaise

2 thick slices of Cheat's Sourdough (see page 10)

1 avocado, halved, peeled and pitted

1 teaspoon lemon juice

extra virgin olive oil, for drizzling

salt and pepper

Mix the mustard and mayonnaise together in a small bowl, toast the bread, then spread the mustard mixture over the toast.

Put one half of the avocado on each slice of toast, mash with the back of a fork and drizzle with a tiny bit of lemon juice.

Season with salt and pepper and drizzle generously with olive oil before serving.

PEANUT BUTTER & BLUEBERRIES

SERVES 1

This delicious combination barely needs a recipe.

crunchy peanut butter

Cheat's Sourdough (see page 10)

handful of blueberries

maple syrup (optional)

Spread crunchy peanut butter liberally over freshly toasted sourdough bread and top with blueberries. For an extra treat, drizzle with a little maple syrup.

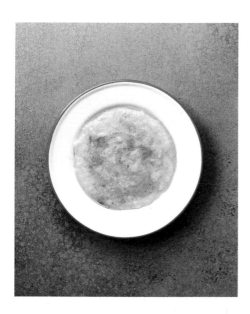

PORRIDGE

This is perhaps the ultimate broke breakfast. Making porridge with water instead of milk is just as delicious and prevents any scorching or sticking to the base of the pan. Just remember that by volume you need to use a 1:3 ratio – 1 cupful of oats to 3 of water. Feel free to add a splash of milk at the end of cooking to loosen the porridge, if you like. It is wonderful eaten just as it is, but try adding 1 tablespoon of cocoa powder for chocolate porridge, or serving it with jam or fruit compote, or topping with fresh fruit.

SERVES 2

50 g (2 oz) rolled oats
  or porridge oats
450 ml (¾ pint) water
pinch of salt
maple syrup or golden
  syrup, to serve

Put the oats and measured water into a high-sided saucepan and set over a medium heat. Add the salt and bring to the boil. Once boiling, reduce the heat to a bare simmer and cook for 10–15 minutes, stirring occasionally, until the oats are tender and cooked through. The porridge should be thick, but still oozy.

Serve warm with golden syrup or maple syrup. Or you can simply sprinkle with sugar.

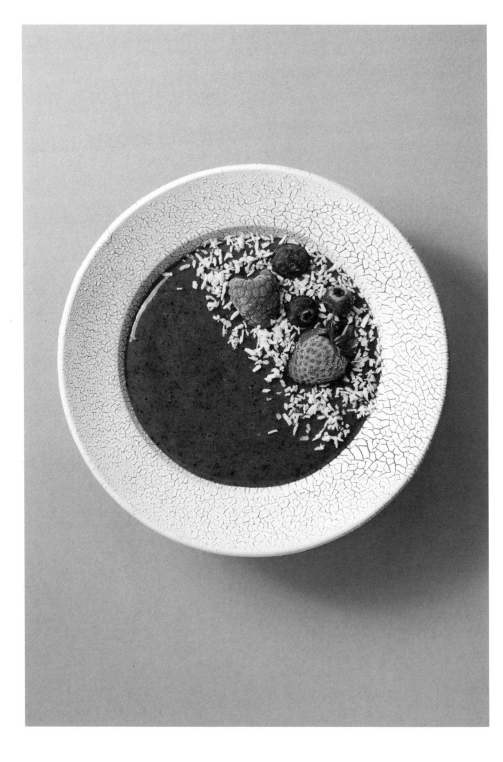

FROZEN FRUIT SMOOTHIE BOWL

Buying pre-packaged frozen fruit works out a lot cheaper than the fresh stuff. You can also freeze your own berries and bananas when they're looking a little past their best, then throw them straight into a blender for a quick, thick morning smoothie bowl. To freeze bananas, peel them, then slice them or leave them whole. Lay them – well spaced apart – on a baking tray until frozen solid, then transfer to a freezerproof container or bag. Freeze berries in the same way, to stop them clumping together.

SERVES 2

2 frozen bananas (see recipe
   introduction)
400 g (13 oz) frozen berries,
   plus extra to serve
2 tablespoons unsweetened
   desiccated coconut

Put all the frozen fruit in a blender and blitz until smooth and thick.

Pour the smoothie into 2 bowls. Serve topped with extra frozen berries and sprinkled with coconut.

BANANA PANCAKES

This is a basic springboard recipe for pancakes that uses just three simple ingredients. You will need a blender to make them but, if you don't have one, use self-raising flour instead of oats – the pancakes won't have the same depth of flavour but they'll still hit the spot. Try adding a pinch of ground cinnamon or nutmeg, a splash of vanilla extract or instant coffee powder, or dousing in maple syrup or melted chocolate afterwards...the variations are endless. It's not necessary to use any cooking fat if you have a nonstick pan, but if you're worried about the pancakes sticking, use a teaspoon of flavourless oil or vegan margarine when frying them.

MAKES 5–6 SMALL PANCAKES / SERVES 2

1 large banana, saving a few
  slices to serve
100 ml (3½ fl oz) dairy-free
  milk
75 g (3 oz) rolled oats
maple syrup, to serve
  (optional)

Put all the ingredients in a blender or food processor and blitz until smooth. The batter should be thicker than double cream.

Preheat a nonstick frying pan over a medium-low heat and add small ladlefuls of batter. Cook each pancake for 2–3 minutes, turning once, until slightly golden on both sides and cooked through.

Serve with the reserved slices of banana and maple syrup, if you like.

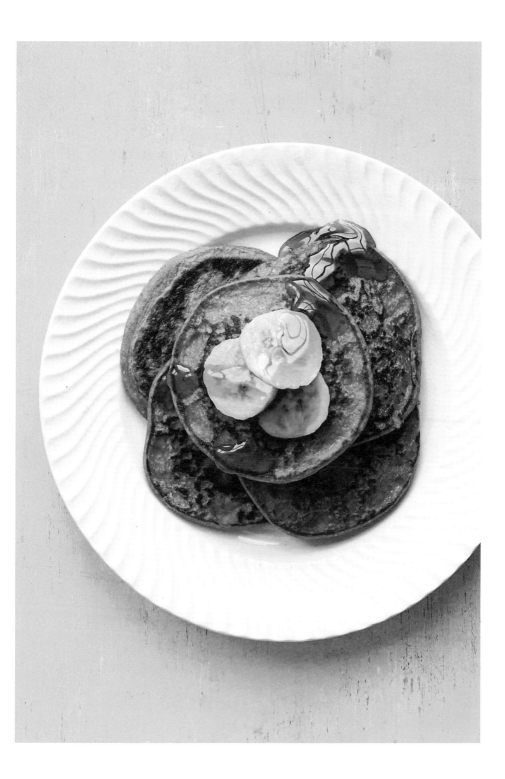

ANY BERRY MUFFINS

These are great for using up any odds and ends of fruit punnets that you have left lying around. Try adding a pinch of ground cinnamon, or the finely grated zest of a lemon, for an extra hit of flavour. These muffins keep in an airtight container for up to 7 days and are the perfect portable breakfast.

MAKES 12

75 ml (3 fl oz) flavourless oil, plus extra for greasing

250 ml (8 fl oz) dairy-free milk

1 teaspoon apple cider vinegar or white wine vinegar

1 teaspoon vanilla extract (optional)

150 g (5 oz) caster sugar or light brown sugar

350 g (11½ oz) self-raising flour

1 teaspoon bicarbonate of soda

1 teaspoon fine sea salt

250 g (8 oz) berries (strawberries, raspberries, blueberries or blackberries, or a mixture of these)

3 tablespoons demerara sugar, for sprinkling (optional)

Preheat the oven to 180°C (350°F), Gas Mark 4 and line a muffin tray with muffin cases. If you don't have cases, you can simply grease the muffin tray, or use squares of nonstick baking paper pressed in as liners.

Put the wet ingredients in a small bowl and whisk well to combine.

In a large bowl, mix the sugar, flour, bicarbonate of soda and salt. Gradually add the wet ingredients to the bowl, whisking well to combine, until you have a smooth batter.

Fold in the berries, then divide the batter evenly between the muffin cases. Sprinkle with demerara sugar, if using, then bake for 14–16 minutes until well risen and golden brown. A skewer inserted into a muffin should come out with no wet batter stuck to it.

Leave to cool on a wire rack, then store in an airtight container.

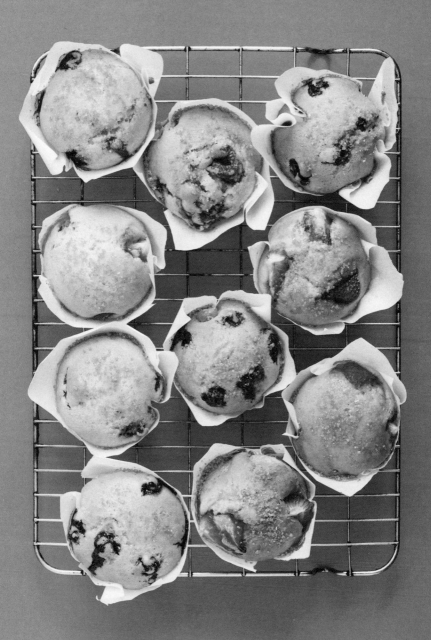

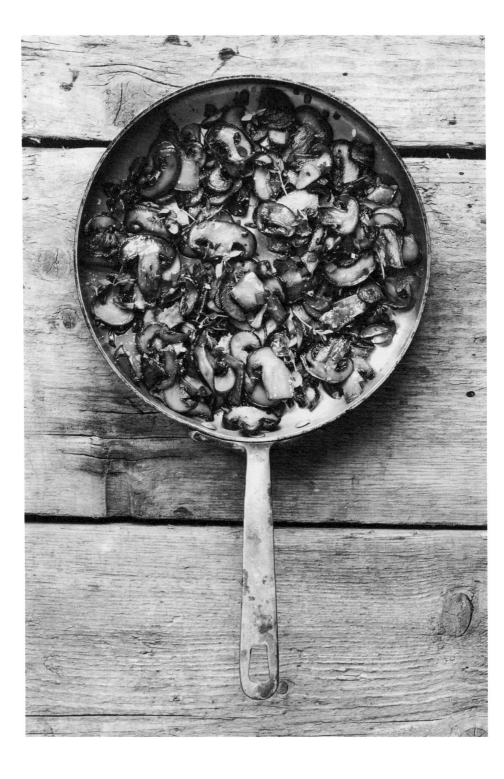

CHILLI GARLIC MUSHROOMS

The trick to cooking really delicious mushrooms is to fry them either in batches or in a big enough pan so that they can turn really golden and caramelized. It is nearly impossible to burn a mushroom, so don't be afraid to get the pan nice and hot – the rest of the flavourings are added after the mushrooms are fully cooked to prevent that bitter, burned garlic taste. Feel free to omit the chilli here or swap the thyme for parsley. Mushrooms are great vehicles for flavour, so use whatever you have to hand.

SERVES 2

3 tablespoons olive oil
300 g (10 oz) chestnut
    mushrooms, finely sliced
2 garlic cloves, finely sliced
1 red chilli, deseeded and
    finely chopped
leaves from 3 thyme sprigs
salt and pepper

Preheat a large frying pan over a medium-high heat and add the olive oil. Fry the mushrooms for 3–4 minutes on each side until deeply golden.

Once you are happy that your mushrooms have enough colour, add the garlic, chilli and thyme and cook for 1 minute until fragrant.

Season well with salt and pepper, then serve with toast, if you like, or as part of a full cooked breakfast.

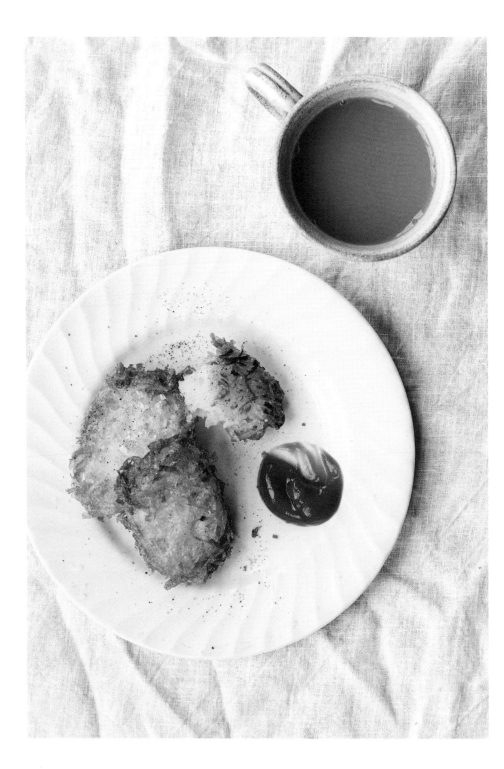

HASH BROWNS

These perfect hash browns only use three ingredients: potatoes, cornflour and oil. You can add 1 teaspoon of onion powder to get that traditional fast food flavour if you like, but they're also delicious without. The method does take a little while, but the results are worth it.

MAKES 8

500 g (1 lb) floury potatoes, peeled
50 g (2 oz) cornflour, plus extra if needed
flavourless oil, for frying
salt and pepper
tomato ketchup, to serve

Use the coarse side of a grater to grate the potatoes into a bowl of very cold water, then leave for 30 minutes, or up to 2 hours, to allow the potatoes to release any starch.

Drain and rinse the grated potato, then bring a saucepan of water to the boil. Drop in the grated potato and blanch for 3–4 minutes – this helps the hash browns to be extra fluffy inside.

Drain and rinse the potato again under cold water, then place in a clean tea towel. Wring out the majority of the liquid – this will allow the hash browns to get crispy edges. You still want a little moisture clinging to the potato strands though, to allow you to shape them.

Tip the potato into a bowl, stir in the cornflour and season well with salt and pepper. The mixture may look dry at first but, when you shape them, the potato will release more moisture.

Shape into 8 hash browns using your hands, sprinkling over more cornflour if the mix is too wet and won't hold together.

Heat enough oil for frying in a deep-sided frying pan, about 2.5 cm (1 inch) deep, over a medium heat. Carefully fry the hash browns for 5–6 minutes on each side until golden. Serve immediately with an extra sprinkling of salt and some tomato ketchup.

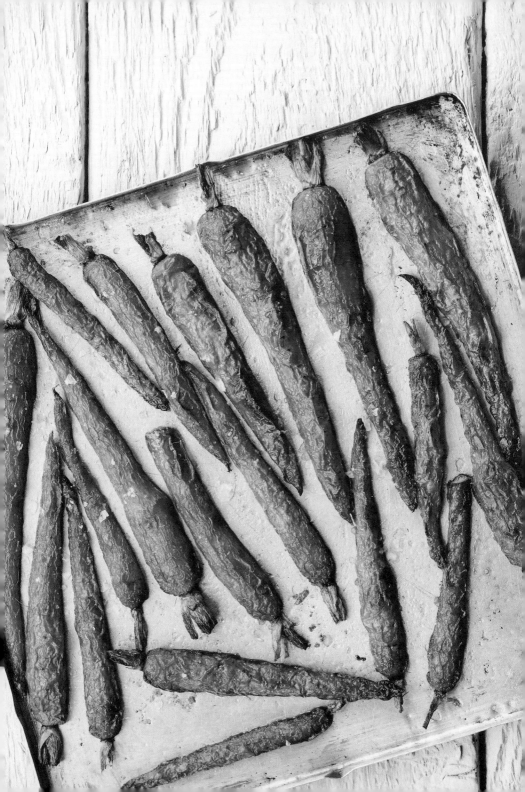

BATCH COOKING

MAPLE ROAST CARROTS

Carrots are one of the cheapest vegetables out there and roasting them brings out their wonderfully sweet flavour, which gets a helping hand here from a splash of maple syrup to make them sticky and moreish. They keep really well, so if you roast a bunch of carrots, you can use them in meals for the rest of the week. If you can get your hands on carrots with tops, then use the leafy greens to make a zero-waste pesto (see page 31). You can leave out the maple syrup and try using any herbs and spices you have in the cupboard if you prefer; for instance, carrots work really well with cumin, paprika and turmeric. (See photo on page 26.)

SERVES 4

1 bunch of carrots, preferably with green leafy tops (total weight about 1 kg / 2 lb), peeled and halved
2 tablespoons olive oil
2 tablespoons maple syrup
salt and pepper

Preheat the oven to 190°C (375°F), Gas Mark 5.

Toss the carrots with the olive oil on a large baking tray and spread them out in an even layer – you want to roast them, not steam them, so they need space to caramelize. Season with salt and pepper and roast for 30–35 minutes until golden and soft to the touch.

Drizzle over the maple syrup and return to the oven for 5 minutes, until the carrots are sticky and smell fragrant.

Enjoy warm, or leave to cool, then store in an airtight container in the refrigerator for up to 5 days.

HARISSA BEAN MASH & ROASTED CARROTS

SERVES 2

400 g (13 oz) can butter
    beans or other white beans
2 tablespoons olive oil
finely grated zest and juice
    of 1 lemon
1 tablespoon harissa
½ quantity Maple Roast
    Carrots (see opposite)
small handful of coriander,
    finely chopped, to serve
salt and pepper

A white bean mash is a great alternative to mashed potatoes, jazzed up here with a dash of harissa spice. Swap in any other canned white beans if you don't have butter beans.

Pour the can of beans, with its liquid, into a small, deep saucepan. Bring to a simmer, then add the olive oil, lemon juice and harissa and mash well with a fork, or use a hand blender to get it super creamy and smooth. You can add a splash of water if you want it to be a bit looser.

Spoon the mash in to a serving dish, top it with the carrots and lemon zest, season well and sprinkle with coriander.

CARROT DHAL

SERVES 4–6

Dhal
½ quantity Maple Roast
    Carrots (see opposite)
1 tablespoon flavourless oil
2 onions, finely chopped
4 garlic cloves, crushed
20 g (¾ oz) fresh root ginger,
    peeled and grated
300 g (10 oz) red lentils,
    washed and drained
1 teaspoon ground turmeric
1 litre (1¾ pints) water
2 tablespoons lemon juice
salt and pepper

Tadka
1 tablespoon flavourless oil
1 teaspoon coriander seeds
1 teaspoon cumin seeds
1 teaspoon black mustard
    seeds

This is a wonderfully comforting Indian-spiced lentil stew that will keep in the refrigerator for up to 4 days. Any left over can be used in Carrot Lentil Fritters (see page 61).

Roughly chop half the roast carrots and set aside.

Heat the oil in a large saucepan. Add the onions and a pinch of salt and cook for 8–10 minutes until soft and translucent. Add the garlic and ginger and cook for 2 minutes more.

Tip in the lentils, turmeric and roughly chopped carrots. Stir to combine, then pour in the measured water. Bring to the boil, then reduce the heat and simmer for 25–30 minutes until the lentils are tender, stirring occasionally.

In a small saucepan or frying pan, heat the oil for the tadka and fry the spices until the mustard seeds pop and everything smells fragrant.

Season the dhal with lemon juice, salt and pepper and stir through the toasted tadka spices. Top the dhal with the remaining whole carrots and enjoy.

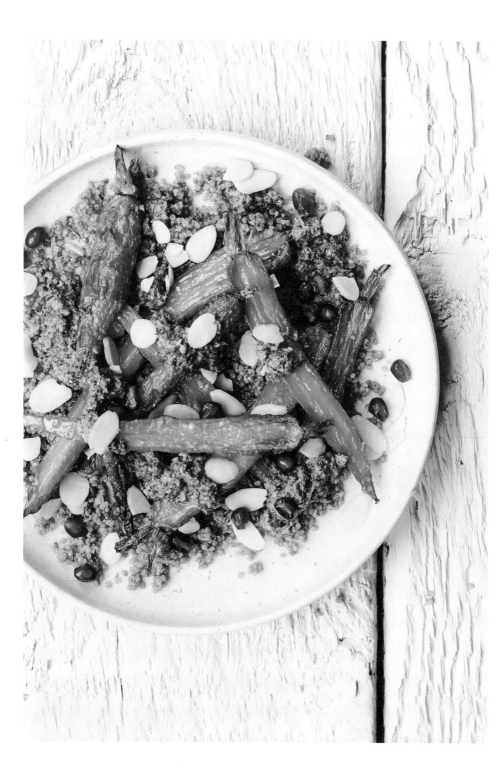

CARROT TOP PESTO & COUSCOUS SALAD

This recipe makes use of the leafy greens on top of bunched carrots that are typically thrown away. If your carrots didn't come with any, use spinach or any other soft leafy greens, or extra herbs, in their place. The pesto has a Middle Eastern flavour with plenty of kick. Swap the couscous here for rice, bulgur wheat, quinoa or any other grain you have on hand.

SERVES 2

Carrot top pesto

1 bunch of carrot tops

large handful of flat leaf
    parsley

large handful of coriander

5 tablespoons olive oil, or
    any flavourless oil

3 tablespoons water, plus
    extra if needed

1 teaspoon ground cumin

1 teaspoon ground coriander

1 green chilli, deseeded and
    roughly chopped

Couscous salad

200 g (7 oz) couscous

2 tablespoons olive oil

finely grated zest and juice of
    1 lemon

½ quantity Maple Roast
    Carrots (see page 28)

40 g (1½ oz) flaked almonds

handful of pomegranate
    seeds (optional)

salt and pepper

Blitz all the ingredients for the pesto in a blender or food processor until fully combined. Add a splash more water if it seems too thick.

Place the couscous in a heatproof bowl with just enough boiling water to cover. Cover the bowl and set aside for 5 minutes to absorb the water.

Fluff up the couscous with a fork, season with salt and pepper and the olive oil, lemon zest and juice.

Top the couscous with the carrots, drizzle with the pesto and scatter with flaked almonds and pomegranate seeds, if using.

MUSHROOM & CAULIFLOWER BOLOGNESE

Deeply satisfying and with an incredible depth of flavour, this recipe works well with other vegetables too; swap the cauliflower for all mushrooms, or try adding lentils to bulk it out. The recipe works well without the carrot and celery, though they do add flavour, and you can leave out the red wine and simply add more water or stock.

SERVES 8

3 tablespoons extra virgin olive oil or regular olive oil

750 g (1½ lb) chestnut mushrooms

1 cauliflower, leaves removed, broken into florets and stalk chopped

1 red onion, finely chopped

1 carrot, finely chopped (optional)

1 celery stick, finely chopped (optional)

3 garlic cloves, finely chopped

2 flat leaf parsley sprigs, roughly chopped, plus extra leaves to serve

100 ml (3½ fl oz) red wine (optional, see recipe introduction)

2 tablespoons tomato purée

400 g (13 oz) can chopped tomatoes or tomato passata

400 ml (14 fl oz) vegan stock

1 tablespoon balsamic vinegar or red wine vinegar

500 g (1 lb) spaghetti, cooked

salt and pepper

Heat the oil in a large casserole dish or large, deep saucepan. Blitz the mushrooms in a food processor until finely chopped – but be careful not to make them into a mushy purée – then transfer to the casserole dish or pan and cook over a medium-high heat until golden brown, about 5 minutes.

While the mushrooms cook, add the cauliflower to the food processor and pulse until the mixture resembles rice. Set aside.

Add the onion, carrot and celery, if using, to the mushroom mixture and cook for a further 8–10 minutes until everything is soft. Add the garlic and parsley sprigs and cook for 1 minute until fragrant.

Add the wine to the pan, if using, and let it bubble up and almost disappear, stirring with a wooden spoon to help deglaze any golden crust on the base of the pan.

Add the tomato purée, chopped tomatoes or passata and stock. Bring to the boil, then reduce the heat and simmer for 15–20 minutes until the sauce has reduced and thickened. Add the cauliflower and cook for a final 10 minutes.

Season with the vinegar, salt and pepper. Serve with cooked, drained spaghetti, with a little parsley sprinkled on top.

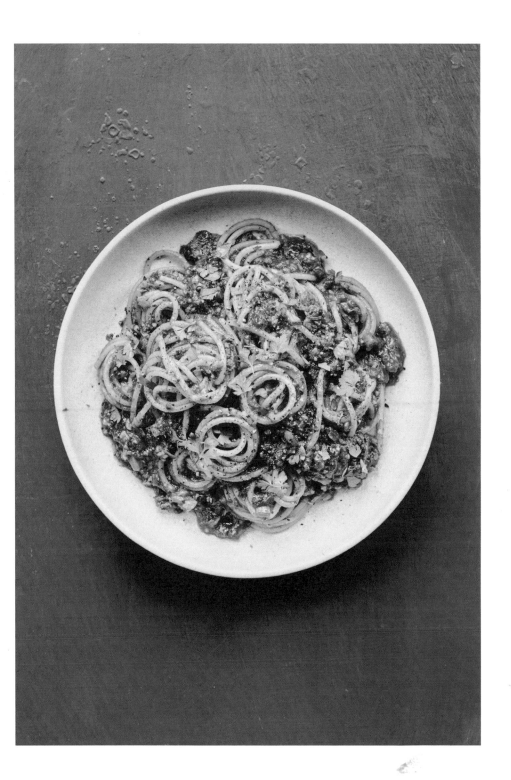

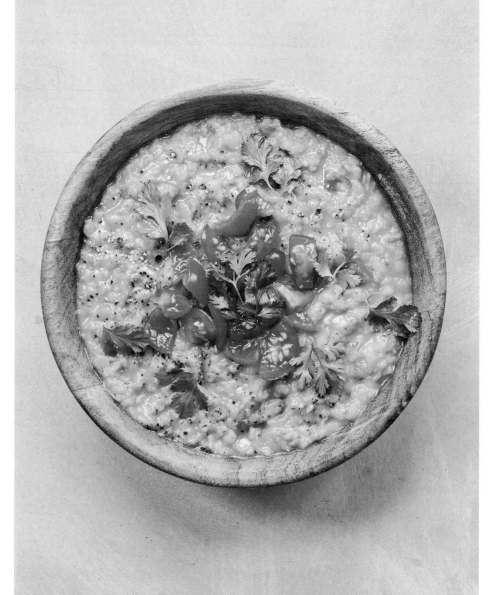

BUDGET HOME-STYLE DHAL

A basic dhal that is great topped with a little roughly chopped tomato and coriander. If you're really struggling for cash you can leave out the ginger, coriander and tomatoes and it will still be just as delicious. This recipe does not include a tadka (freshly toasted whole spices in oil served on top) – if you'd like to add that, fry whole coriander seeds, cumin seeds, mustard seeds and fresh curry leaves in a little flavourless oil for 1 minute until fragrant. Try adding coconut milk in place of the water, use different lentil varieties, throw in some finely chopped chillies or stir through some spinach at the end...dhal is the perfect dish to experiment with.

SERVES 6

1 tablespoon flavourless oil

2 onions, finely chopped

4 garlic cloves, crushed

large handful of coriander, stalks finely chopped, leaves reserved to garnish

20 g (¾ oz) fresh root ginger, peeled and grated

1 teaspoon ground turmeric

1 teaspoon garam masala

300 g (10 oz) red lentils, washed and drained

2 tomatoes or a handful of cherry tomatoes, roughly chopped

1 litre (1¾ pints) water or vegan stock

2 tablespoons lemon juice

salt and pepper

Heat the oil in a large saucepan. Add the onions and a pinch of salt and cook for 8–10 minutes until soft and translucent. Add the garlic, coriander stalks and ginger and cook for 2 minutes more.

Add the turmeric and garam masala and cook for 1 minute until fragrant.

Tip in the lentils and half the tomatoes. Stir to combine, then pour in the measured water or stock.

Bring to the boil, then reduce the heat and simmer for 25–30 minutes until the lentils are tender, stirring occasionally.

Season the dhal with the lemon juice and salt and pepper. Top with the remaining chopped tomato and the coriander leaves. This will keep in the refrigerator for up to 4 days and also freezes well.

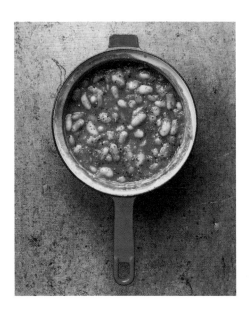

DIY BAKED BEANS

One of the quickest dishes you can make and it beats a canned version any day!

SERVES 6

1 tablespoon flavourless oil

1 shallot, finely chopped

1 large garlic clove, crushed

2 x 400 g (13 oz) cans cannellini beans, or other white beans, drained and rinsed

250 ml (8 fl oz) tomato passata

200 ml (7 fl oz) water or vegan stock

1 tablespoon caster sugar, or to taste

1–2 tablespoons apple cider vinegar, or to taste

salt and pepper

Heat the oil in a medium saucepan over a medium-low heat. Add the shallot and cook for 6–8 minutes until soft and translucent, then add the garlic and cook for 1 minute.

Add the beans, passata and measured water or stock and bring to the boil. Reduce the heat to a bare simmer, add the sugar and vinegar and cook for 10–15 minutes until the sauce has reduced slightly.

Taste and adjust the seasoning accordingly, adding more sugar or vinegar depending on your preference.

WHOLE-CAN TANGY BLACK BEANS

This dish is zero waste, using all the goodness from the can to render the sauce creamy, unctuous and thick. Sweet and savoury, it is the ultimate convenience food: since canned beans require no soaking or long cooking, you can make it in an instant. Serve in Sweet Potato Quesadillas (see page 76) or with tacos (see page 99) or over chips for a loaded-fries situation. Or simply top with chopped avocado and a bit of coriander and serve with tortilla chips.

SERVES 6

2 tablespoons olive oil

1 onion, finely chopped

3 garlic cloves, finely
   chopped

2 x 400 g (13 oz) cans
   black beans

400 ml (14 fl oz) water
   or vegan stock

½ teaspoon ground cumin

½ teaspoon ground coriander

½ teaspoon smoked paprika

1 tablespoon caster sugar

1 tablespoon apple cider
   vinegar

salt and pepper

Heat the oil in a large frying pan. Add the onion and garlic and cook for 6–8 minutes over a medium heat until softened.

Add the beans and their liquid to the pan, then add the water or stock to the cans and swirl to make sure you loosen every last drop before adding that too.

Season with the spices, sugar and salt and pepper. Stir well and cook for 15 minutes over a medium heat, stirring occasionally, until thickened. Use your spatula to smash some of the beans, to help to thicken the mixture, or use a hand blender to blitz half the beans roughly.

Take the pan off the heat, stir in the vinegar and season to taste. The beans will thicken further as they cool.

Eat immediately, or store in the refrigerator in an airtight container for up to 5 days. This freezes well; just make sure it's fully cooled before freezing.

CONFIT TOMATOES

A great way to use up any wrinkly, forgotten tomatoes and to make yourself a delicious flavoured oil using the cheapest base oil that you can get your hands on. The tomatoes keep for ages and you can use their garlicky, rich oil any time you're making a savoury base – in marinara sauce (see page 89) or in Mushroom & Cauliflower Bolognese (see page 32), for example. The measurements here are just a guide – you don't need to make this much or you can make more. All you need is some tomatoes in a snug-fitting container with enough oil to come halfway up their sides. Eat as a topping on toast or pizza (see page 91), add to a salad or reheat as a quick pasta sauce.

FILLS A 1 KG (2 LB) JAR

750 g (1½ lb) tomatoes, halved
1 garlic bulb, halved
a few thyme, oregano, basil or rosemary sprigs (optional)
350–500 ml (12–17 fl oz) olive oil
salt and pepper

Preheat the oven to 120°C (250°F), Gas Mark ½.

Put the tomatoes into a snug-fitting, deep baking tray, placing them cut sides up as this stops the liquid from the tomatoes leaching into the oil. Add the halved garlic bulb, preferably placing it cut side down so it infuses the oil with more garlic flavour. Season well and add the herbs, if using.

Pour the olive oil over the tomatoes until it reaches halfway up the sides of the tray, then pop them in the oven for 1½–2 hours until the whole house smells amazing and the tomatoes have shrivelled and softened.

Allow to cool. Meanwhile, sterilize a jar by cleaning it thoroughly in hot soapy water, then putting it in a moderate oven preheated to 150°C (300°F), Gas Mark 2 for 10 minutes to dry. Rubber jar seals should not go in the oven; instead, place them in a bowl and cover with boiling water to sterilize.

Decant the cooled tomatoes into the sterilized jar. They will keep well at room temperature for up to 1 month.

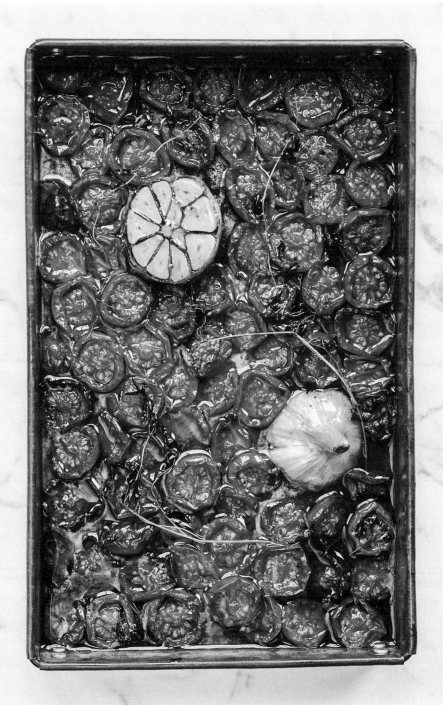

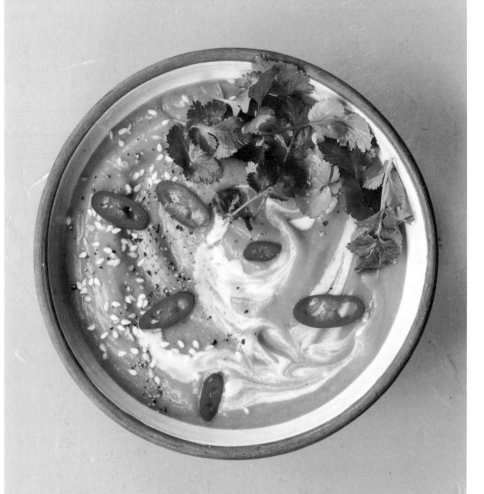

SPICED SQUASH SOUP

This wonderfully warming butternut soup is a low-effort, high-reward dish. It freezes really well in individual portions or keeps in the refrigerator for up to 4 days.

SERVES 8

2 tablespoons flavourless oil

1 large red onion, roughly sliced

3 garlic cloves, roughly sliced

25 g (1 oz) fresh root ginger, peeled and roughly chopped

1 tablespoon mild curry powder

3 tablespoons vegan bouillon powder

1 litre (1¾ pints) water

1 large butternut squash (about 1 kg / 2 lb), peeled, deseeded and roughly chopped

200 g (7 oz) can coconut milk, 2 tablespoons reserved to garnish

2–3 tablespoons lime juice

salt and pepper

To serve

1 red chilli, deseeded and finely sliced

large handful of coriander, roughly chopped

2 tablespoons sesame seeds

In a large saucepan or casserole dish, preheat the oil over a medium heat. Fry the onion for 6–8 minutes until golden and starting to soften. Add the garlic and ginger and fry for 2 minutes, then add the curry powder, stir well and cook for 1 minute.

Add the bouillon powder with the measured water and the squash chunks. Bring to the boil, then reduce the heat to a simmer and cover with a lid. Cook for 1 hour, until the squash is tender when pierced with a fork.

Add the coconut milk and use a hand blender to blitz the soup until smooth, or allow to cool and use a food processor or blender.

Season with the lime juice, salt and pepper, swirl in the reserved coconut milk and serve with the red chilli slices, coriander and sesame seeds, either scattered on top or in bowls on the side for people to help themselves to.

SWEET POTATO & CAULIFLOWER CURRY

A sweeter take on the traditional Indian dish of aloo gobi, which is made from regular potatoes and cauliflower. Serve with rice, naan bread or on its own. Feel free to swap the sweet potatoes for carrots, or the spinach for any leafy greens, such as kale or cabbage.

SERVES 8

3 tablespoons flavourless oil
2 onions, finely sliced
25 g (1 oz) fresh root ginger, peeled and finely grated
5–6 garlic cloves, finely sliced
1 tablespoon mild curry powder
1 teaspoon ground turmeric
2 sweet potatoes (total weight about 750 g / 1½ lb), peeled and cut into 2.5 cm (1 inch) cubes
500 ml (17 fl oz) vegan stock
400 g (13 oz) can coconut milk
1 large cauliflower, broken into small florets and stalk finely chopped
300 g (10 oz) spinach
2 tablespoons lemon juice
1 red chilli, deseeded and finely chopped

Heat the oil in a large, heavy-based saucepan over a medium heat. Add the onions and cook for 10 minutes until soft and translucent. Add the ginger and garlic and cook for 2 minutes more.

Add the curry powder and turmeric and stir constantly, cooking for 1 minute.

Tip in the sweet potatoes and the stock. Bring to the boil, then reduce the heat and simmer for 15 minutes until the sweet potato is almost tender. Add the coconut milk and cauliflower and cook for a final 10 minutes.

When the curry is almost ready, add the spinach to wilt. Season with lemon juice, salt and pepper and scatter in the chilli. Serve with a sprinkling of coriander, if you like.

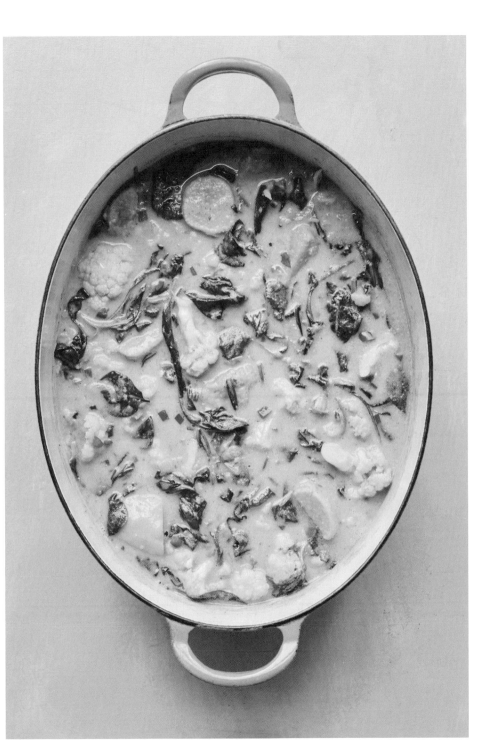

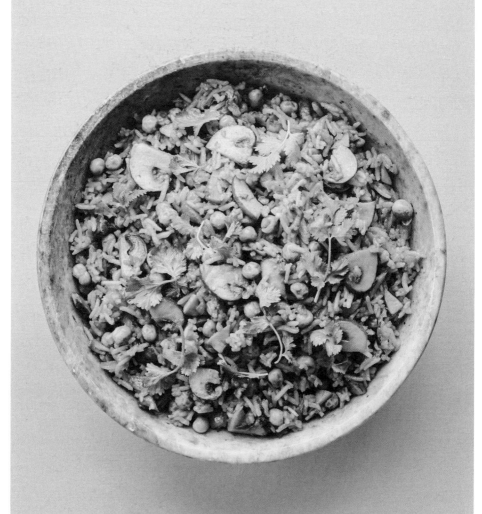

VEGETABLE PILAU RICE

*Serve this with Sweet Potato & Cauliflower Curry (see page 42) or
roasted vegetables. It's also fantastic refried in a pan with some oil
for a quick fried rice dish.*

SERVES 8

2 tablespoons flavourless oil

2 onions, finely chopped

400 g (13 oz) mushrooms,
    roughly chopped

4 garlic cloves, finely
    chopped

300 g (10 oz) basmati rice,
    washed thoroughly

1 teaspoon salt

1 tablespoon ground turmeric

400 ml (14 fl oz) vegan stock

200 g (7 oz) frozen peas

large handful of coriander,
    roughly chopped, to serve

Heat the oil in a large saucepan over a medium heat. Fry
the onions for 8–10 minutes until soft and translucent.

Add the mushrooms and cook for 5–6 minutes until
golden; they may give off some moisture, so keep going
to drive that off and cook them until they are starting to
brown. Now tip in the garlic and cook for a final 2 minutes.

Pour in the rice, salt and turmeric and stir for 2–3 minutes
to toast the rice.

Slowly add the stock, then place a tea towel on top of
the pot, followed by a lid, lifting the corners of the towel
up and over the lid to keep them away from the flames.
Reduce the heat to as low as it will go and cook for
15 minutes.

After 15 minutes, tip the peas on top of the rice, replace the
tea towel and lid and cook for a final 5 minutes.

Turn off the heat and leave to stand for 5 minutes before
serving. Fluff up the rice with a fork, evenly distributing the
peas as you do so. Serve with a scattering of coriander.

BAKED POTATOES

Bake at least 4 potatoes at a time to save on fuel costs and keep them in the refrigerator ready to make into loaded baked potatoes.

MAKES 8

8 large baking potatoes, such as Maris Piper or King Edward
a little flavourless oil (optional)
salt (optional)

Preheat the oven to 180°C (350°F), Gas Mark 4.

Prick the potatoes all over with a knife or fork. If you like your potatoes to have a crunchy exterior, rub them all over with oil, then sprinkle with salt.

Roast in the oven for 1–2 hours, depending on size, until tender all over when gently squeezed. If you're in a hurry, try microwaving the potatoes for 7–8 minutes, then finishing them off in the oven for 15 minutes instead.

LOADED INDIAN POTATOES

SERVES 2

2 large potatoes, baked (see above)
200 g (7 oz) frozen peas, defrosted
2 teaspoons garam masala, chaat masala or curry powder, plus extra to serve
large handful of coriander, finely chopped
½ red onion, finely chopped
1 tomato, finely chopped
¼ cucumber, finely chopped

Limey cashew cream
100 g (3½ oz) unsalted cashew nuts, soaked in cold water overnight or soaked in boiling water for 1 hour
4 tablespoons lime juice
salt and pepper

A fancy way to enjoy a baked potato, with a subtle warmth and a crunchy kachumber-style cucumber salad on top.

Preheat the oven to 180°C (350°F), Gas Mark 4.

Make the limey cashew cream: drain and rinse the soaked cashews, then blitz in a food processor with 3 tablespoons of lime juice and a few splashes of water until you have a smooth, creamy sauce. Season to taste and set aside.

Split the potatoes in half, keeping them attached at the base. Scoop out the majority of the potato inside and transfer to a bowl. Add the peas and garam masala, chaat masala or curry powder and most of the coriander, saving some to serve. Season with salt and pepper, then spoon the mixture back into the potato skins and bake for 10–15 minutes until piping hot.

Meanwhile, mix the red onion, tomato and cucumber with the remaining lime juice and season with salt and pepper.

Spoon the limey cashew cream on top of the baked potatoes followed by the crunchy vegetable salad. Sprinkle with the remaining coriander and a little garam masala to serve.

LOADED POTATOES WITH CHUNA SWEETCORN

SERVES 2

Smashed chickpeas with the right flavourings deliver a salty, briney punch in this veganized version of a classic tuna sweetcorn, aka 'chuna sweetcorn'.

400 g (13 oz) can chickpeas
1 tablespoon Dijon mustard
2 tablespoons tahini
finely grated zest and juice
    of 1 lemon
2 spring onions, finely sliced
1 tablespoon capers in brine
large handful of flat leaf
    parsley, finely chopped
165 g (5½ oz) can sweetcorn,
    drained
2 large potatoes, baked,
    reheated if necessary
    (see opposite)
salt and pepper

Empty the chickpeas and their liquid into a small, deep saucepan. Bring to the boil and cook for 10–15 minutes until the chickpeas are extremely tender.

Drain and transfer to a bowl. Mash the chickpeas with the back of a fork and then add all the remaining ingredients except the potatoes, seasoning to taste with salt and pepper.

Split the potatoes in half, keeping them attached at the base. Load the chuna sweetcorn into the middle of the potato, with plenty of extra on top, then serve.

LOADED POTATOES WITH SMOKY SPICY BEANS

SERVES 2

Unlocking the potential of your spice drawer can transform basic baked beans into something complex and warming. This variation would be wonderful with a side of corn on the cob, for that proper barbecue feel.

½ quantity DIY Baked Beans
    (see page 36)
2 teaspoons smoked paprika
1 teaspoon ground cumin
½ teaspoon cayenne pepper
2 large potatoes, baked,
    reheated if necessary
    (see opposite)
small handful of chives, finely
    chopped
salt and pepper

Put the beans in a saucepan and stir in the spices. Bring to the boil, then reduce the heat to a simmer for 5 minutes. Season to taste.

Split the potatoes in half, keeping them attached at the base. Load with the spicy beans and top with a sprinkling of chives, then serve.

CHILLI CON VEGGIE

This gently spicy, incredibly hearty stew is great served over rice or used to load fries. You can really add whatever vegetables you have to hand; some finely chopped carrot, aubergine, courgette or red pepper would bulk it out further. You could also use any kind of bean here: cans of mixed beans are great, or swap out half the kidney beans for black beans, or make a white bean chilli con veggie instead.

SERVES 8-10

3 tablespoons extra virgin olive
   oil or regular olive oil
500 g (1 lb) chestnut
   mushrooms, finely chopped
1 large onion, finely chopped
1 celery stick, finely chopped
3 garlic cloves, finely chopped
   or crushed
1 red chilli, finely chopped,
   deseeded if you prefer
   less heat
2 teaspoons ground cumin
2 teaspoons ground coriander
1 teaspoon smoked paprika
2 tablespoons vegan bouillon
   powder
1 teaspoon caster sugar
2 x 400 g (13 oz) cans chopped
   tomatoes
2 x 400 g (13 oz) cans red
   kidney beans, drained
   and rinsed
salt and pepper

To serve (optional)
1-2 avocados, halved, peeled,
   pitted and finely sliced
coriander sprigs
lime wedges

In a large casserole dish or saucepan, heat the oil over a medium heat. Add the mushrooms and cook for 5-6 minutes until golden.

Add the onion and celery and cook for a further 10 minutes until translucent and soft. Add the garlic and chilli and cook for 1 minute, then add the ground spices and cook for 1 minute until fragrant.

Add the vegan bouillon powder, sugar and tomatoes. Bring to the boil, then reduce the heat to a simmer for 20-30 minutes until the sauce has begun to reduce. Add the beans and cook for a further 10 minutes, then taste and adjust the seasoning. Serve with avocado slices, coriander and lime wedges, if you like.

This will keep in the refrigerator for 4 days or, in portions, in the freezer for up to 6 months.

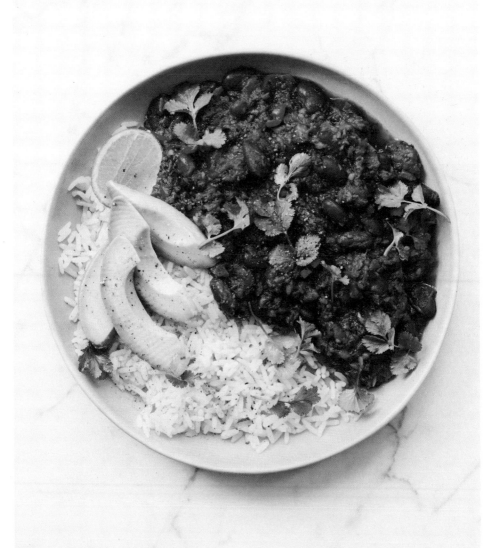

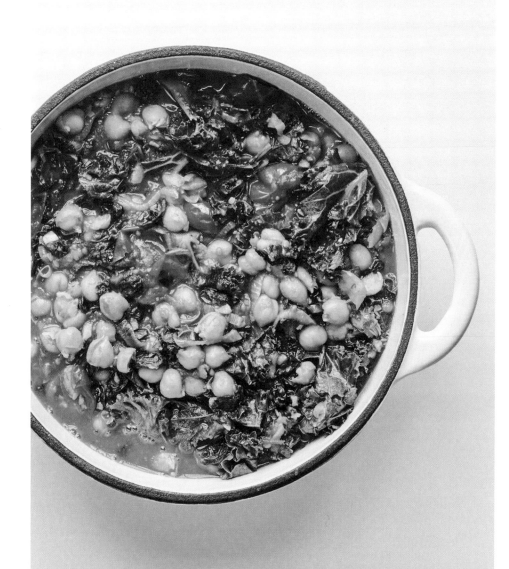

CHICKPEAS & GREENS

This autumnal Mediterranean dish is sweet, tangy and wonderful mopped up with crusty bread or served over couscous. If you plan to freeze it in small batches, do so before adding the greens; wilt these in only once the stew has defrosted and been reheated, to retain their nutritive value and bright colour.

SERVES 6-8

3 tablespoons olive oil
1 large red onion, finely sliced
2 garlic cloves, finely
   chopped or crushed
1 teaspoon sweet paprika
½ teaspoon ground cumin
½ teaspoon ground cinnamon
2 x 400 g (13 oz) cans
   chickpeas
400 g (13 oz) can chopped
   tomatoes
400 g (13 oz) leafy greens,
   such as kale, chard or
   spinach, coarse ribs
   removed
50 g (2 oz) raisins or sultanas
salt and pepper

Heat the oil in a large, heavy-based saucepan. Add the onion and cook it, without browning, over a medium-low heat for 8–10 minutes until soft and translucent.

Add the garlic and cook for 2 minutes, then add the spices and cook for a further 1 minute.

Tip in the chickpeas and their liquid as well as the chopped tomatoes. Bring to the boil, then reduce the heat to a simmer for 20 minutes until reduced and thickened.

Add the greens (unless you plan to freeze the stew – see recipe introduction) and raisins and season well. Cook for 5–10 minutes more until the greens are wilted and cooked through. Taste and adjust the seasoning. Scatter with plenty of parsley, if you like, and serve.

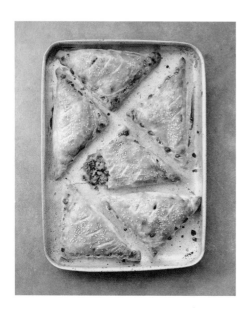

CURRIED LEEK & POTATO PUFFS

These Indian-spiced curry puffs are ideal to take on a picnic or for a packed lunch.

MAKES 6

½ **quantity Roasted Leeks &**
   Potatoes (see opposite)
75 g (3 oz) frozen peas,
   defrosted
1 tablespoon lemon or lime
   juice
1 tablespoon curry powder
500 g (1 lb) block of vegan
   puff pastry
a little plain flour, for dusting
2 tablespoons dairy-free milk
1 tablespoon sesame seeds
salt and pepper

Preheat the oven to 190°C (375°F), Gas Mark 5.

In a medium-sized bowl, lightly mash the roasted leeks and potatoes, leaving some large chunks. Fold in the peas, lemon or lime juice and curry powder. Season and set aside.

On a lightly floured surface, roll out the puff pastry into a large square (about 35 cm / 14 inch). Cut it in half, then cut each half into 3 to give 6 rectangles. Roll each rectangle out a little more to give you a squarer shape of thinner pastry.

Heap 1–2 tablespoons of filling in the centre of each pastry square and fold one corner in diagonally over the filling, making a triangular-shaped pasty. Using your finger or a pastry brush, put some dairy-free milk on the seam to help you to seal it, push gently with your fingers, then crimp with your fingers or a fork to seal tightly.

Repeat with the remaining pastry squares and filling, then brush all over with dairy-free milk and sprinkle with sesame seeds.

Bake on a large baking tray for 30–35 minutes until puffed and deep golden. Serve warm or at room temperature.

These will keep in the refrigerator for up to 3 days.

ROASTED LEEKS & POTATOES

MAKES 4 PORTIONS

1 kg (2 lb) floury potatoes, peeled and cut into 2.5 cm (1 inch) cubes
2 leeks, thoroughly washed and thickly sliced
3 tablespoons olive oil
salt and pepper

Two of the cheapest vegetables out there, these deceptively simple flavours are the perfect base for so many things. If you'd rather not roast the leeks and potatoes, you can cook them in a frying pan instead.

Preheat the oven to 170°C (340°F), Gas Mark 3½ .

Toss the potatoes and leeks with the oil on a large baking tray and season well. Roast for 30–40 minutes until golden and soft.

Enjoy hot or store in an airtight container in the refrigerator for up to 5 days.

ROASTED LEEK & POTATO SOUP

SERVES 2

½ quantity Roasted Leeks & Potatoes (see above)
1 garlic clove, finely sliced
leaves from 2–3 thyme sprigs
400 ml (14 fl oz) vegan stock
small handful of chives, finely chopped
salt and pepper

This really couldn't be easier to pull together – plus it freezes very well for soup emergencies.

Put the leeks and potatoes, the garlic, thyme and stock in a large, deep saucepan. Bring to the boil, then reduce the heat and simmer for 10 minutes.

Use a hand blender to purée the soup until silky smooth, or allow to cool, then blend in a blender or food processor. Season with salt and pepper to taste.

Reheat if necessary and serve sprinkled with chopped chives and pepper.

VERY VERSATILE DIY FALAFELS

Soaking your own dried chickpeas and fava beans overnight is totally worth it and makes for a more traditional, firmer falafel. If you make them with canned chickpeas, the texture is a lot mushier. If you can't find fava beans – which are dried broad beans – just swap them for some extra chickpeas. The mixture freezes really well – simply freeze it just before you add the baking powder, then, after defrosting, stir in the baking powder and continue as instructed. You can also shape the mixture into patties to make falafel burgers if you prefer.

MAKES 30

400 g (13 oz) dried
    chickpeas
150 g (5 oz) fava beans or
    dried broad beans
large handful of coriander
large handful of flat leaf
    parsley
large handful of spinach
    (about 50 g/2 oz)
1 red onion, peeled and
    quartered
3 garlic cloves, peeled
2 teaspoons ground cumin
2 teaspoons ground
    coriander
finely grated zest and juice
    of 1 lemon
1 tablespoon baking powder
flavourless oil, for deep-
    frying
salt and pepper

Place the chickpeas and fava beans in a very large bowl and cover generously with cold water. Leave overnight to soak; they will double in size.

The next morning, drain and rinse them well and put them in a food processor with the herbs, spinach, onion and garlic. Blitz until fully combined but still with some crumbly texture.

Tip the mixture out into a large bowl and add the ground spices, lemon zest and juice. Season to taste. If you're making the falafel straight away, add the baking powder (this should always be the last step before shaping to ensure you get lovely puffy and light falafel).

Shape the mixture into balls or pucks, using around 2 tablespoons of mixture for each.

Heat enough oil for frying in a deep saucepan, about 3.5 cm (1½ inches) deep, over a medium-high heat until the oil shimmers. Carefully add the falafel in batches, 5–6 at a time, and fry for 6–8 minutes, turning regularly to get an even, deep golden-brown colour. Drain on kitchen paper, season with salt and keep warm to enjoy hot or allow to cool to room temperature.

Store in an airtight container in the refrigerator for up to 5 days.

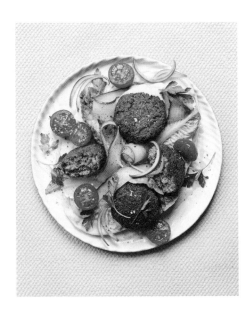

OPEN FALAFEL PITTAS

SERVES 4

1 red onion, finely sliced
1 tablespoon red wine
    vinegar
1 teaspoon caster sugar
4 pitta breads or flatbreads
1 quantity Any Can Hummus
    (see page 115)
12 Very Versatile DIY Falafels
    (see opposite)
small handful of Little Gem
    lettuce leaves
½ cucumber, shaved
12 cherry tomatoes, halved
flat leaf parsley sprigs
salt and pepper

Falafel and hummus are partners in crime. The quick pickled red onions will keep in the refrigerator for a week, ready to add a nice tang to lacklustre dishes.

In a small bowl, mix the red onion with the vinegar, sugar and a pinch of salt. Scrunch together with your hands and leave for at least 20 minutes before serving.

Toast the pitta breads or flatbreads, then top with the hummus, falafels, lettuce, cucumber and tomatoes. Sprinkle with the parsley and quick pickled red onion before serving.

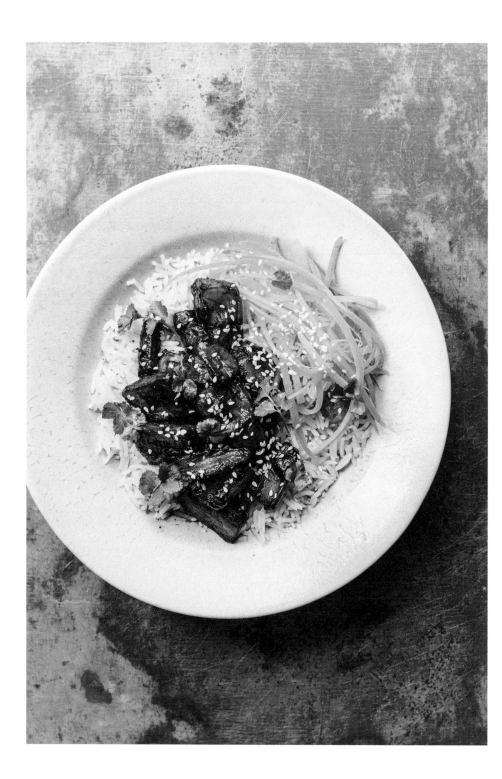

STICKY SWEET AUBERGINES

*The miso paste gives an incredible depth of flavour to this dish, but the
best thing about these aubergines is how soft and rich they are from
being peeled and fried; they act like sponges for the sauce. Make a big
batch, scaling up depending on how many aubergines you have, then
serve them over rice, stirred into noodles or as part of a salad bowl.*

SERVES 4

flavourless oil, for
   deep-frying
2 large aubergines, peeled
   and cut into small wedges
6 tablespoons miso paste
4 tablespoons soy sauce
2 tablespoon caster sugar
2 tablespoon rice wine
   vinegar or lime juice

To serve
white rice
grated carrot
sesame seeds
small handful of coriander,
   roughly chopped

Preheat the oven to 200°C (400°F), Gas Mark 6.

Heat enough oil for frying in a saucepan, about 5 cm
(2 inch) deep, over a medium-high heat until the oil
shimmers. Add the aubergines, in batches, and cook for
10–12 minutes until golden and softened.

Meanwhile, whisk together the miso, soy sauce, sugar and
vinegar or lime juice, then pour on to a baking tray.

Use a slotted spoon to remove the aubergines from the
hot oil and place straight on the baking tray. Toss the
aubergines in the sauce, then bake for 10 minutes until the
sauce has become sticky and caramelized.

Serve immediately with white rice and grated carrot, and
sprinkled with sesame seeds and coriander, or store in an
airtight container in the refrigerator for up to 3 days.

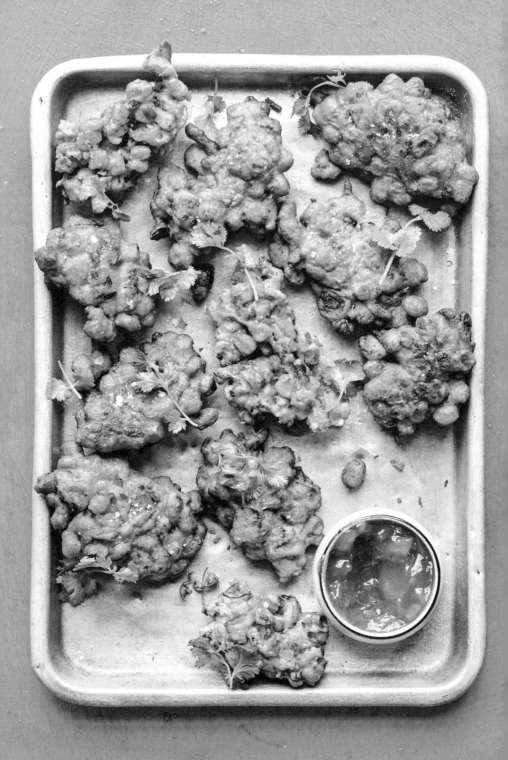

READY IN 20

ANY VEGETABLE BHAJI

One of the best ways to make cheap vegetables go further, taste more delicious and satisfy a crowd is to deep-fry them in a crunchy coating. It's not rocket science. Once you've mastered bhaji batter, you can fry any sturdy-ish vegetables. Try thinly sliced onion, carrot, courgette, broccoli, kohlrabi, cauliflower, Brussels sprouts, kale... you name it. They will work mixed together or you can be a purist about it. You can even "bhaji" old herb stems and salad leaves. The possibilities are endless.

SERVES 4

200 g (7 oz) gram (chickpea)
    flour
175 ml (6 fl oz) warm water
small handful of coriander,
    very finely chopped
1 small green chilli, deseeded
    and very finely chopped
1 teaspoon ground turmeric
1 teaspoon ground cumin
1 teaspoon chilli powder
flavourless oil, for
    deep-frying
500 g (1 lb) vegetables of
    your choice, finely sliced
salt and pepper

Put the gram flour into a large bowl. Add most of the measured water and whisk well to combine. You may not need all of the water – add just enough to give a batter the consistency of double cream.

Whisk in the coriander, chilli and ground spices and season well with salt and pepper.

Heat the oil in a large saucepan over a medium heat, filling the pan no more than half full, until the oil shimmers.

Dip the sliced vegetables in the batter, stir, then lower spoonfuls of them carefully into the hot oil. Fry in batches, for a few minutes, turning regularly to get an even golden-brown colour.

Remove with a slotted spoon and drain on kitchen paper. If some of the batter has come away from the bhajis, simply fish it out and serve with the bhajis. Eat the bhajis hot, with mango chutney, if you like.

CARROT LENTIL FRITTERS

SERVES 4

250 g (8 oz) / about 1 serving
    Budget Home-style Dahl
    (see page 35)
50 g (2 oz) gram (chickpea)
    flour
1 large carrot, peeled and
    grated
small handful of coriander,
    chopped
2 spring onions, finely sliced
finely grated zest and juice
    of 1 lime
flavourless oil, for
    deep-frying
salt and pepper

These make good use of leftover dhal. Use this recipe as a blueprint and try stirring through grated courgette, wilted spinach or any leftover vegetables.

Mix the dhal with the gram flour, carrot, coriander and spring onions, then season with the lime zest and juice and some salt and pepper.

Heat 2.5 cm (1 inch) of oil in a large frying pan. When the oil shimmers, spoon in ladlefuls of the thick batter, and use the back of the ladle to spread each into a patty shape.

Cook for 3–4 minutes on each side until golden brown. Remove with a slotted spoon and drain on kitchen paper. Serve hot, while you cook the remaining fritters.

SWEETCORN & ONION PAKORAS

SERVES 4

300 g (10 oz) sweetcorn
4 spring onions, finely sliced
1 green chilli, deseeded and
    finely chopped
large handful of coriander,
    finely chopped, plus extra
    to serve
1 tablespoon garam masala
100 g (3½ oz) plain flour or
    gram (chickpea) flour
1 teaspoon salt, plus extra
    to serve
mango chutney, to serve
    (optional)

The gentle spice is wonderful in these miniature crispy pakoras. If you don't have a green chilli or any coriander, just add ½ teaspoon each of chilli powder and ground coriander. (See photo on page 58.)

Mix the sweetcorn, spring onions, chilli, coriander, garam masala, flour and salt in a large bowl. Stir together, adding 2–3 tablespoons of water until the batter is just wet enough to cling together.

Heat 3.5 cm (1½ inches) of oil in a large saucepan over a medium heat until the oil shimmers. Spoon tablespoonfuls of the thick batter directly into the oil in batches, 4–5 at a time, and cook for 3–4 minutes until golden brown.

Drain on kitchen paper, then serve hot, with an extra sprinkling of salt and coriander, and mango chutney, if you like, while you cook the remaining pakoras.

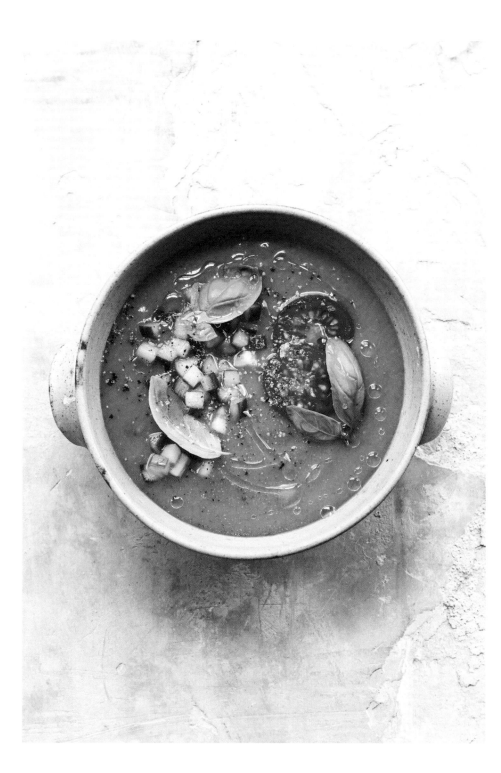

FOOLPROOF GLORIOUS GAZPACHO

This is simply summer in a bowl and, with no cooking required, you can stay cool in the kitchen. Pick up a bargain at your local greengrocer or farmers' market, plumping for those tomatoes that are a bit squished and ugly (it's all getting blitzed together anyway). This silky-smooth soup is best served chilled, so it's good to put it in the refrigerator for at least 1 hour before serving, or pop in a few ice cubes before eating, if you run out of time.

SERVES 8-10

875 g (1¾ lb) tomatoes, roughly chopped

1 red pepper, cored, deseeded and roughly chopped

1 small red onion, quartered

1 garlic clove, peeled

1 cucumber, roughly chopped

1 stale slice of bread (about 125 g/4 oz)

2 tablespoons sherry vinegar or red wine vinegar, or to taste

2 tablespoons caster sugar, or to taste

2 tablespoons extra virgin olive oil or regular olive oil, plus extra for drizzling

salt and pepper

To serve (optional)
¼ cucumber, finely chopped
small handful of cherry tomatoes, sliced
small handful of basil leaves

In a large blender, or in a large bowl with a hand blender, blitz all the soup ingredients together, seasoning well with salt and pepper. Taste and add more sugar or vinegar depending on the sweetness of your tomatoes – you're looking for a sharp and sweet soup with a slight spicy burn from the garlic.

You can eat the soup as is, or pass it through a sieve to get a smoother result.

Refrigerate before serving sprinkled with salt and pepper and drizzled with olive oil, or with chopped cucumber, sliced tomatoes and basil leaves.

COURGETTE SATAY

These vegetable skewers are really versatile – try replacing the courgette with aubergine, sweet potato or any squash. The sauce will appear to split after first mixing it but, after flashing it in the microwave, it should come together. If you don't have skewers, just griddle or fry the courgettes.

SERVES 2

Skewers
2 courgettes, cut into 3 cm (1¼ inch) chunks
1 teaspoon ground turmeric
1 tablespoon soy sauce
1 tablespoon sesame oil or flavourless oil

Satay sauce
3 tablespoons crunchy peanut butter
5 tablespoons coconut milk
1 tablespoon soy sauce
1 tablespoon caster sugar
1 tablespoon lime juice

To serve
carrot shavings
cucumber slices
thinly sliced red onion
1 red chilli, deseeded and finely sliced
small handful of coriander, roughly chopped
small handful of mint leaves

Soak 6 bamboo skewers in water to prevent them burning later on.

Preheat a large griddle or frying pan. In a bowl, toss the courgettes with the turmeric, soy sauce and oil. Lay them out in a single layer in the pan and cook for 3–4 minutes on each side until caramelized and soft.

Meanwhile, whisk together the satay sauce ingredients and microwave on high for 30 seconds to help it come together smoothly, then stir.

Serve the skewers with lots of fresh crunchy salad – carrot, cucumber, red onion and red chilli – with coriander and mint scattered over and the satay sauce in a bowl on the side.

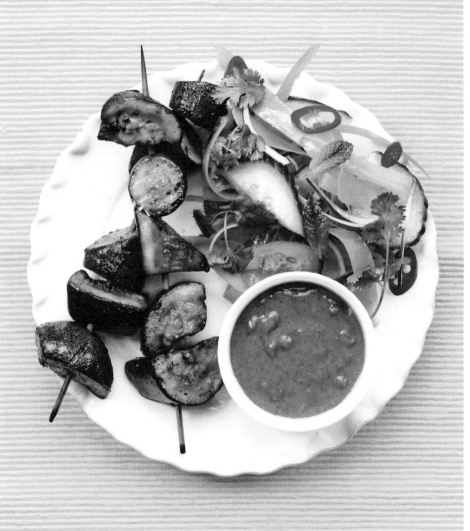

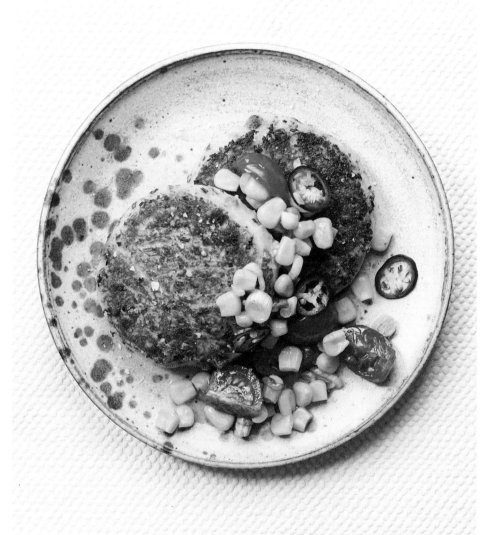

BACK-OF-THE-FRIDGE FRITTERS

The perfect meal when all you have in the refrigerator are some old herbs and spring onions, and a few frozen peas in the freezer. (It's an extra bonus if you already have some leftover mashed potato.) You can add any leftover vegetables you have lying around, such as broccoli, greens or grated carrot, and the fritters also work really well with mashed sweet potato instead of regular potato. The tomato and sweetcorn salsa gives them a Mexican twist, but they're just as delicious on their own served with some hot sauce.

SERVES 3–4

Fritters

1–2 large baking potatoes, peeled and roughly chopped, or 2 portions of leftover mashed potato

200 g (7 oz) frozen peas, defrosted

large handful of chives, finely chopped

large handful of coriander, finely chopped

2–3 spring onions, finely sliced

flavourless oil, for frying

salt and pepper

Sweetcorn salsa

100 g (3½ oz) cherry tomatoes, roughly chopped

100 g (3½ oz) sweetcorn

1 green chilli, deseeded and finely sliced

1 spring onion, finely sliced

finely grated zest and juice of 1 lime

1 tablespoon olive oil

If you don't have any leftover mash, put the chopped potato into a pan of cold water and bring to the boil. Cook for 8–10 minutes until soft. Drain in a colander, then mash with a fork or pass through a potato ricer into a large bowl.

Add the peas, chopped herbs and spring onions and season well. Shape the mixture into 6–8 patties, depending how large you want them.

Heat 1 cm (½ inch) of oil in a large frying pan. Fry the potato fritters on each side for 3–4 minutes, in batches if you need to, so as not to crowd the pan. Try not to move them around too much – you want them to develop a crust and they can be quite delicate.

Meanwhile, mix all the ingredients for the salsa together in a small bowl.

Serve the fritters warm with the salsa on the side, making sure you get plenty of the limey tomato juice from the bottom of the bowl.

5 SIMPLE DRESSINGS

BASIC VINAIGRETTE

½ shallot, finely chopped
2 tablespoons vinegar (white wine vinegar, red wine vinegar or apple cider vinegar)
1 tablespoon Dijon mustard
3 tablespoons extra virgin olive oil or regular olive oil
1–2 teaspoons maple syrup or sugar
salt and pepper

A basic vinaigrette is a foundation dressing that any cook should have in their arsenal. It's a great way of learning how to balance the acidity, saltiness and sweetness: the ratios of vinegar to oil to sweetener will vary depending on the brand or type of ingredient you're using, so taste regularly until you're happy that the dressing is delicate, sharp, ever so slightly sweet and salty.

Whisk together the shallot, vinegar and mustard. Slowly drizzle in the oil, whisking constantly until the vinaigrette has thickened and emulsified.

Season to taste with maple syrup or sugar, salt and pepper.

MAPLE MUSTARD DRESSING

4 tablespoons olive oil
2 tablespoons white wine vinegar
1 tablespoon maple syrup
1 tablespoon wholegrain mustard
1 teaspoon Dijon mustard
salt and pepper

An equivalent to a honey-mustard dressing, that just happens to saves the bees.

Whisk all the ingredients together and season with salt and pepper to taste.

MISO SESAME DRESSING

2 tablespoons flavourless oil
2 tablespoons sesame oil
1 tablespoon lime juice
1 tablespoon miso paste
1 tablespoon soy sauce
1–2 teaspoons maple syrup
  or sugar
salt and pepper

Great tossed with warm roasted vegetables – they soak up lots of the savoury flavour – and good over raw spinach and cucumber, served as a cooling side dish.

Whisk all the ingredients together and season with salt and pepper to taste.

JALAPEÑO & LIME DRESSING

2 tablespoons finely chopped
  pickled jalapeños
finely grated zest and juice
  of 1 lime
2 tablespoons flavourless oil
2 tablespoons finely chopped
  coriander
1–2 teaspoons maple syrup
  or sugar
salt and pepper

If you have a half-eaten jar of pickled jalapeños lingering in the refrigerator, make a batch of this dressing and toss it through a sweetcorn and black bean salad, or serve over a simple tossed salad with lettuce and avocado for an instant hit of Mexican flavour.

Whisk all the ingredients together and season with salt and pepper to taste.

GARLIC & CHIVE VINAIGRETTE

2 tablespoons red wine
  vinegar
1 garlic clove, finely chopped
1 tablespoon finely chopped
  chives
3 tablespoons extra virgin
  olive oil or regular olive oil
1–2 teaspoons maple syrup
  or sugar
salt and pepper

Wonderful with chopped salads and green vegetables, plus this is also rather nice to use as a dip for your homemade pizza crusts (see page 88).

Whisk together the vinegar, garlic and chives. Slowly drizzle in the oil, whisking constantly until the vinaigrette has thickened and emulsified.

Season to taste with maple syrup or sugar, salt and pepper.

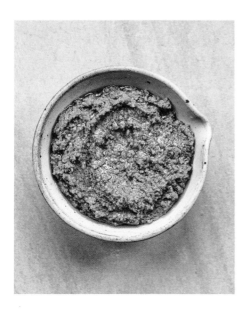

BREADCRUMB PESTO

MAKES 350 G (11½ OZ)

30 g (1¼ oz) breadcrumbs,
  toasted if fresh
30 g (1¼ oz) any raw nuts
  or an extra 30 g (1¼ oz)
  breadcrumbs
large handful of spinach
  (about 40 g/1½ oz)
large handful of basil
  (about 40 g/1½ oz)
finely grated zest and juice
  of 1 lemon
1 garlic clove
4 tablespoons extra virgin
  olive oil
3–4 tablespoons cold water
salt and pepper

The single best thing you can do with leftover herbs is to blitz them into a pesto.

Whizz all the ingredients together in a food processor until smooth, adding as much of the measured water as you need to loosen the pesto. Season with salt and pepper to taste.

Keep in an airtight container in the refrigerator for up to 2 weeks.

CORIANDER & PARSLEY ZHOUG

MAKES 350 G (11½ OZ)

large handful of coriander
(about 40 g/1½ oz)
large handful of parsley
(about 40 g/1½ oz)
large handful of spinach
(about 40 g/1½ oz)
finely grated zest and juice
of 1 lemon
3 tablespoons extra virgin
olive oil or regular olive oil
1 green chilli, seeds left in,
roughly chopped
1 teaspoon ground cumin
1 teaspoon ground coriander
2–3 tablespoons cold water
salt and pepper

Zhoug is a spicy Yemeni pesto. Gorgeously green and fiercely hot, use it to top any roasted vegetables to liven them up and serve alongside something cooling, such as Limey Cashew Cream (see page 46) or cucumber.

Whizz all the ingredients together in a food processor until smooth, adding as much of the measured water as you need to loosen the pesto. Season with salt and pepper to taste.

Keep in an airtight container in the refrigerator for up to 2 weeks.

PEA & MINT PESTO

MAKES 350 G (11½ OZ)

100 g (3½ oz) frozen peas,
blanched in boiling water
for 1 minute, then drained
large handful of mint (about
30 g/1¼ oz)
large handful of spinach
(about 40 g/1½ oz)
finely grated zest and juice
of 1 lemon
3 tablespoons extra virgin
olive oil or regular olive oil
2–3 tablespoons cold water
salt and pepper

Peas are cheaper than buckets of herbs and nuts and they lend a great hearty texture to this pesto, which is lovely alongside spring vegetables, such as asparagus, new potatoes and broad beans.

Whizz all the ingredients together in a food processor until smooth, adding as much of the measured water as you need to loosen the pesto. Season with salt and pepper to taste.

Keep in an airtight container in the refrigerator for up to 2 weeks.

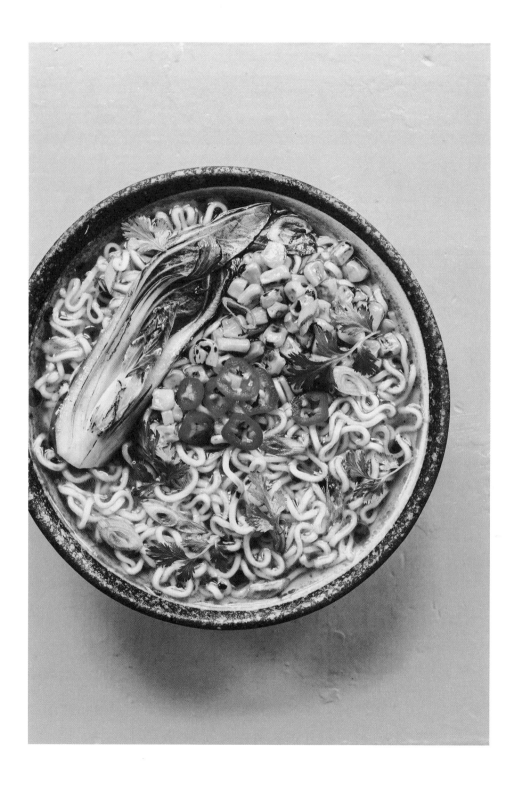

PIMPED INSTANT RAMEN

More instant ramen packets are vegan than you might expect.
This is a speedy and simple lunch. Use any vegetables you have
in the refrigerator – the ingredients below are just a guide.

SERVES 2

2 single-portion packets
    instant ramen noodles
2 tablespoons soy sauce
1 teaspoon chilli oil
1 head of bok choi, halved
    lengthways
100 g (3½ oz) sweetcorn
1–2 spring onions, finely
    sliced
1 red chilli, deseeded and
    finely sliced
small handful of coriander,
    roughly chopped

Cook the ramen noodles according to the packet instructions. Add the soy sauce and chilli oil to the broth and leave to cook for another 2 minutes.

Heat a frying pan over a high heat and char the cut sides of the bok choi halves. Add the sweetcorn and allow to fry until charred and caramelized too.

Top the ramen with the charred bok choi and sweetcorn and sprinkle over the spring onions, chilli slices and coriander before serving.

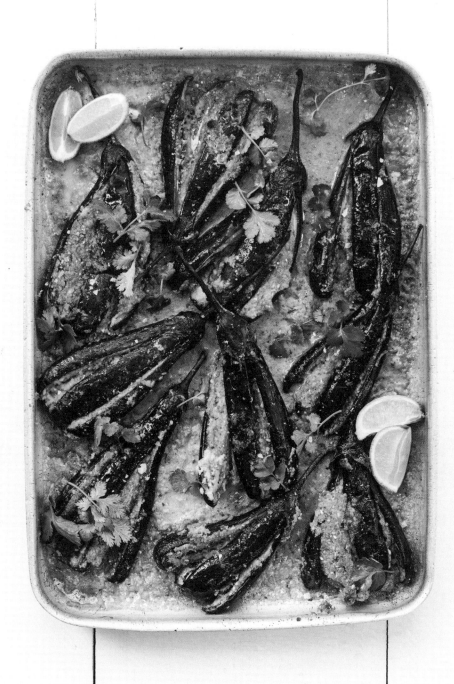

SESAME AUBERGINE CURRY

This curry is quickest to prepare when you use baby aubergines, but you can use regular aubergines if you can't find them. It's a fairly dry curry using a quick nutty paste that you stuff inside the aubergines, which is cooked at a fiercely high heat to get it to your table in 20 minutes. It also works well as a slower-cooked dish if you prefer: cook it at 180°C (350°F), Gas Mark 4 for 35 minutes, covering with foil to prevent the liquid from evaporating. If you'd like it to be saucier, add about 250 ml (8 fl oz) more stock.

SERVES 2

80 g (3¼ oz) raw peanuts
50 g (2 oz) sesame seeds
2 garlic cloves
large handful of coriander,
    stalks finely chopped,
    leaves reserved to garnish
2 tablespoons brown sugar
1 tablespoon curry powder
50 ml (2 fl oz) water, plus
    extra if needed
10 small aubergines,
    quartered, but left intact at
    the stalk end, or 2 regular
    aubergines, cut into small
    wedges
2 tablespoons flavourless oil
400 ml (14 fl oz) vegan stock
1 lime, cut into wedges, to
    garnish
salt and pepper

Preheat the oven to 240°C (475°F), Gas Mark 9.

In a blender or a pestle and mortar, blitz or work together the peanuts, sesame seeds, garlic, coriander stalks, sugar and curry powder with the measured water, adding more to loosen if necessary – you want a spreadable paste.

Lay the aubergines on a large baking tray. Spoon the paste on to the cut sides of the aubergines (or, if using regular aubergines, just toss the wedges in the paste). If you have any curry paste leftover, set it aside. Toss the aubergines in the oil and season well with salt and pepper.

Roast the aubergines for 5–8 minutes until starting to blister and sizzle. Add any remaining curry paste and the stock, stir briefly and cook for a further 10–12 minutes until the aubergine is tender and the sauce has reduced. Serve with lime wedges and coriander leaves.

SWEET POTATO QUESADILLAS

These are honestly miles better than any stringy cheese quesadillas you have ever eaten in the past. The sweet potato has a zesty kick from the lime and the perfect level of spice – completely addictive. Try adding Whole-can Tangy Black Beans (see page 37) or other vegetables into the mix. The method of cooking the quesadillas in semi-circles rather than sandwiching the filling between 2 circles ensures you don't lose any filling when flipping them.

SERVES 2

2 sweet potatoes (total weight 500–600 g/ 1 lb–1 lb 5 oz)
2 tablespoons finely chopped pickled jalapeños
2 spring onions, finely sliced
large handful of coriander, finely chopped
1 lime
2 large tortillas
2 tablespoons flavourless oil
salt and pepper

Prick the sweet potatoes all over with a knife and microwave on high for 5–7 minutes until tender. Cut in half, then scoop out the flesh into a bowl.

Mix the sweet potato flesh with the jalapeños. Add most of the spring onions and coriander, reserving some of both for serving. Finely grate over the zest of the lime, then cut the lime in half and add the juice of half the lime to season the filling. Cut the other half into wedges for serving.

Distribute the filling between the 2 tortillas, heaping it on half of each tortilla, then folding over the empty side and pressing it down to make sure the filling is in an even layer.

Heat the oil in a large frying pan and add the tortillas. Fry for 2–3 minutes on each side until golden brown and the filling is warm inside.

Cut into wedges and serve with the reserved spring onions and coriander, and the lime wedges.

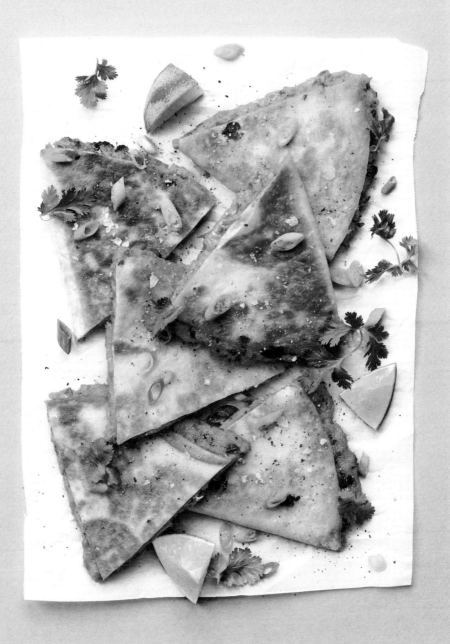

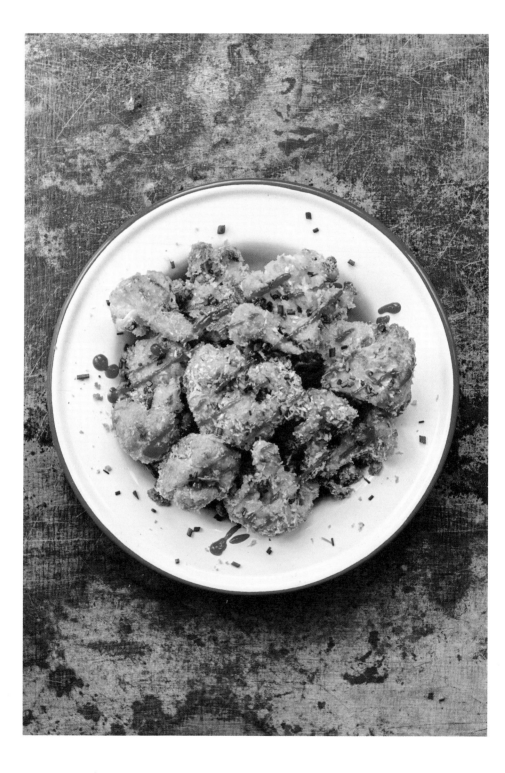

CAULIFLOWER NUGGETS

Irresistibly crunchy and so simple to make – there's no time wasted breadcrumbing the individual cauliflower florets. Mixing the wet ingredients and breadcrumbs on the baking tray means you get lots of extra crispy morsels of flavoured breadcrumb shards to serve with the nuggets. Switch up the spices if you fancy a change – these would be wonderful in a traditional fast-food style with onion and garlic powder or given an Indian twist with garam masala and ground cumin.

SERVES 2

1 medium cauliflower, broken into florets
4 tablespoons cornflour
1 tablespoon smoked paprika
1 teaspoon ground coriander
4 tablespoons dairy-free milk
100 g (3½ oz) panko breadcrumbs or regular very dry breadcrumbs
4 tablespoons flavourless oil
salt and pepper

To serve
small handful of finely chopped chives (optional)
hot sauce

Preheat the oven to 200°C (400°F), Gas Mark 6.

Steam or boil the cauliflower in salted water for 5 minutes until almost tender. Drain well and transfer to a large baking tray.

Sprinkle the cornflour and spices over the florets and toss to coat.

Pour over the dairy-free milk and toss to coat again, followed by the breadcrumbs, tossing a final time to make sure every crevice is covered in breadcrumbs. Season well with salt and pepper.

Drizzle the oil over the breadcrumbed florets and bake for 15 minutes until the breadcrumbs are deeply golden and the cauliflower is cooked through. Serve with chopped chives, if you like, and hot sauce.

CHICKPEA TABBOULEH

Make a double batch of these chickpeas, because on their own they're a great snack and much healthier than crisps. Experiment with different spice combinations or grate in any crunchy vegetables you have around. Stored in an airtight container, the tabbouleh will keep in the refrigerator for up to 1 week.

SERVES 2

400 g (13 oz) can chickpeas, drained and rinsed
1 tablespoon ras al hanout
2 tablespoons olive oil
200 g (7 oz) couscous
1 tablespoon vegan bouillon powder
1 orange, zest finely grated, fruit segmented
1 carrot, grated or julienned
1 cucumber, grated or julienned
½ red onion, finely chopped
6 radishes, finely sliced
large handful of flat leaf parsley, roughly chopped
large handful of coriander, roughly chopped

Preheat the oven to 190°C (375°F), Gas Mark 5.

Dry the drained chickpeas thoroughly, tip on to a baking tray and toss with the ras el hanout and oil. Roast for 10–15 minutes until crisp.

Meanwhile, put the couscous in a large heatproof bowl and stir in the bouillon powder until evenly combined. Pour over just enough boiling water to cover the couscous, then cover the bowl with a plate or clingfilm for 5–8 minutes until the couscous has absorbed all the liquid.

To assemble the tabbouleh, fluff up the couscous with a fork and stir in the orange zest and segments, carrot, cucumber, red onion, radishes and herbs. Top with the crispy chickpeas and enjoy.

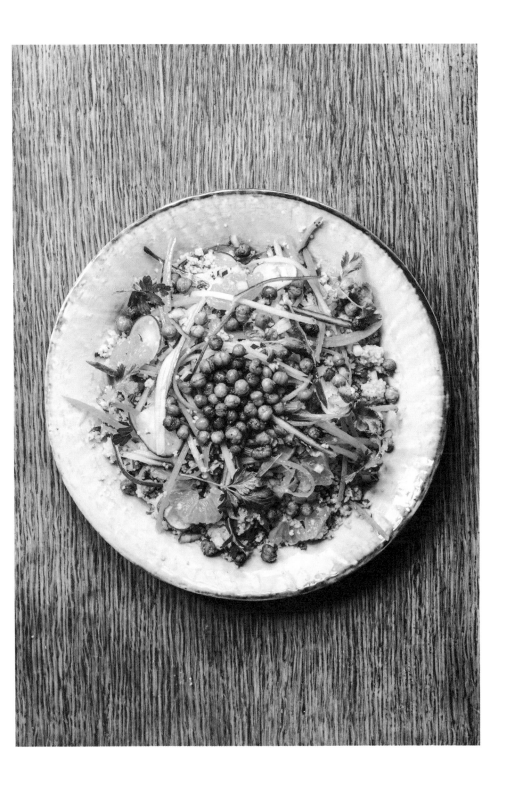

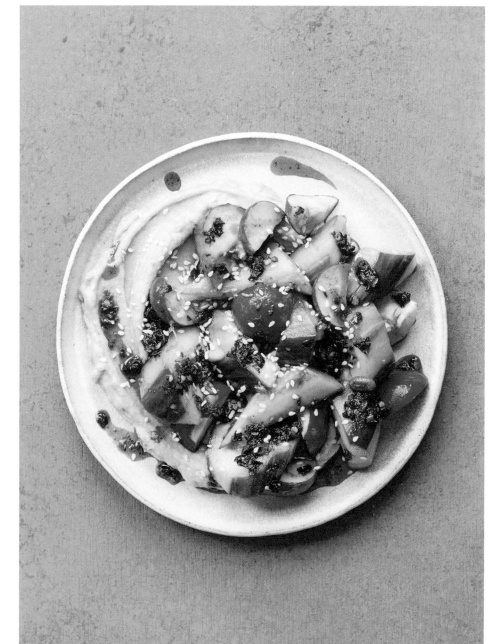

BASHED CUCUMBERS & RADISHES

There is a perfect balance here between cool and spicy. The sharp, tangy avocado serves as a much needed creamy and cooling partner to the crunchy and spicy cucumbers and radishes. This dish is at its best when using a proper Chinese crispy chilli oil, the kind with lots of crunchy bits in.

SERVES 2

1 cucumber, roughly peeled
250 g (8 oz) radishes
2 tablespoons crispy chilli oil, plus extra (optional) for drizzling
2 tablespoons soy sauce
1 tablespoon caster sugar
½ quantity Avocado Crema (optional, see page 114)
sesame seeds, to serve

Use a large knife to roughly chop the cucumbers and halve the radishes, then cover each piece with the flat of the knife and use the heel of your hand to bash down. Place the bashed pieces in a bowl and toss with the chilli oil, soy sauce and sugar.

Spread the Avocado Crema, if using, on a serving plate and top with the bashed cucumbers and radishes and all the sauce. Serve with more chilli oil, if you like things spicy, and sesame seeds.

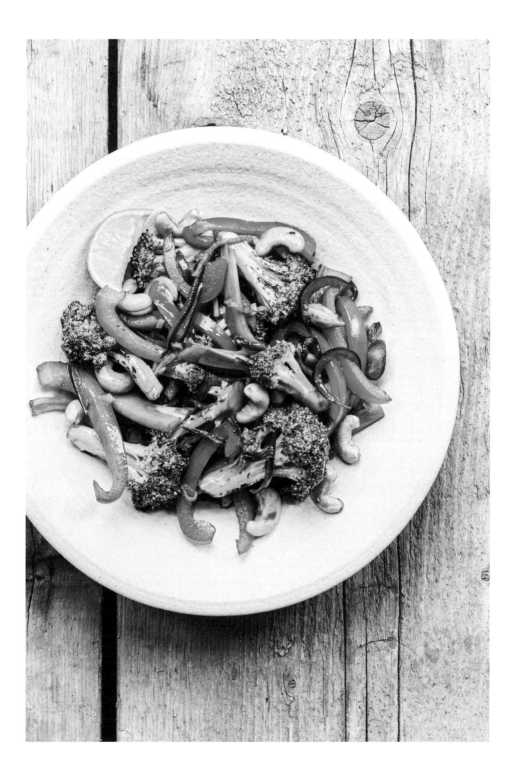

BROCCOLI STIR-FRY

Don't throw your broccoli stalk away! It is great for bulking out this
stir-fry, adds another texture and has a very intense broccoli flavour.
If you don't want to use cashew nuts, simply leave them out.

SERVES 2

2 tablespoons sesame oil
   or flavourless oil
1 red onion, finely sliced
1 garlic clove, finely chopped
   or crushed
20 g (¾ oz) fresh root ginger,
   peeled and grated or
   julienned
1 broccoli head, broken into
   florets, stalk finely sliced
1 red pepper, cored,
   deseeded and finely sliced
50 g (2 oz) cashew nuts
50 ml (2 fl oz) soy sauce
1 tablespoon maple syrup
finely grated zest and juice
   of 1 lime
lime wedges, to serve

Heat the oil in a wok, then add the onion, garlic and ginger and cook over a high heat for 2–3 minutes until golden.

Add the broccoli, red pepper and cashew nuts and stir-fry for 2–3 minutes more until beginning to gain colour and tenderize.

Add the soy sauce, maple syrup and lime zest and juice and cook for 1 minute until the sauce bubbles up and coats all the vegetables. Serve with lime wedges.

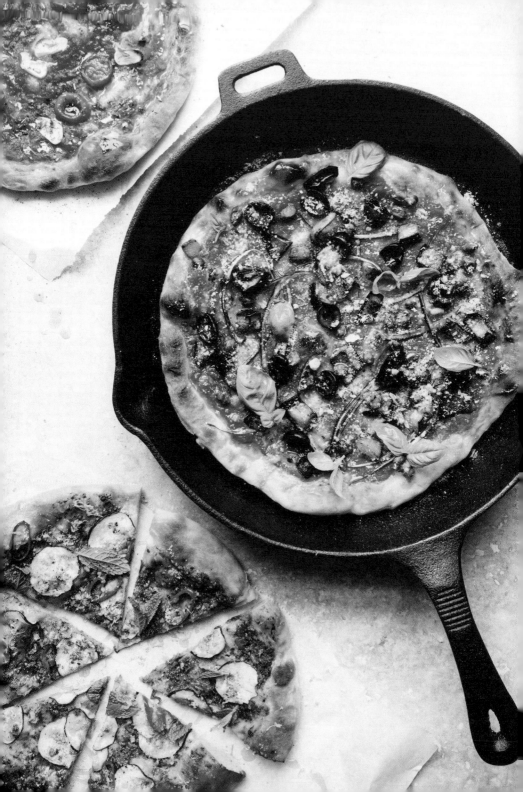

IMPRESS A CROWD

HOMEMADE PIZZA DOUGH

You'll be hard-pressed to find someone who isn't impressed by homemade pizza, and it's one of the cheapest things you could ever make. Get your guests involved in shaping the bases and topping their own pizzas and ensure everyone's up for sharing, because it's hard to make more than one at a time. Make, slice, eat, repeat. This dough recipe is enough for when you have a few friends over, though it also halves and doubles very easily. You're going to need a frying pan or skillet that can go straight from the hob to the oven (no plastic or wood!) to make sure you get a crunchy bottom and a blistered golden top.

MAKES 4 THIN CRUST OR 3 THICK CRUST PIZZA BASES

400 g (13 oz) strong white bread flour
1 teaspoon salt
1 teaspoon fast-action dried yeast
1 tablespoon olive oil, plus extra for oiling
200–250 ml (7–8 fl oz) lukewarm water
2 tablespoons semolina (optional)
toppings of your choice (see pages 89–91)

In a large bowl, combine the flour, salt, yeast and olive oil. Gradually add the measured water until you have a sticky, but not too-wet, dough. Knead on a lightly oiled table – or in the bowl of a stand mixer – until smooth, elastic and springy (this will take 8–10 minutes). Leave the ball of dough in a lightly oiled bowl, covered with a tea towel, until doubled in size (about 1 hour). You can also leave it in the refrigerator overnight for a slower rise.

When you're ready to make your pizzas, preheat the grill to its highest possible setting. Also start to preheat an ovenproof frying pan over a medium-high heat.

Divide the dough into 3 for slightly thicker pizzas or 4 for thin. Roll each piece of dough into a ball, then use either a rolling pin or your hands to push it out into a circle as wide as the base of the pan (probably 20–25 cm/8–10 inches), keeping the edges a little thicker. If your dough resists being stretched, leave it covered with a tea towel for 5 minutes to relax, then come back to it. You shouldn't need any flour on the table to do this, as the dough contains oil.

Sprinkle a little semolina into your frying pan for an extra-crunchy base or leave it out if you don't have any. Carefully place a pizza base in the pan – the pan will be hot.

Add your chosen toppings to your pizza base in the pan – see recipes below and on pages 90–1.

When you're ready, put the pizza on the highest shelf underneath the grill for 5–6 minutes until the toppings are cooked through and the crust is golden and starting to get slightly charred. Repeat to cook the remaining pizzas.

PIZZA MARINARA

SERVES 3–4

Marinara sauce
400 g (13 oz) can whole plum
    tomatoes
½ garlic clove, grated
2 tablespoons tomato purée
salt and pepper

1 quantity Homemade Pizza
    Dough (see opposite)
1 garlic clove, finely sliced
    (optional)
15 cherry tomatoes, halved
    (optional)
pinch of dried oregano
    (optional)
extra virgin olive oil or regular
    olive oil, for drizzling

The simplest, cheapest way to top a pizza, this just happens to be one of the most delicious as well. You'll soon be a big fan of uncooked tomato sauce, as it tastes so fresh when it's flashed in the oven on the pizza base and requires minimal effort. If you have leftover sauce, use it with pasta or in Mushroom & Cauliflower Bolognese (see page 32).

To make the marinara sauce, either squeeze the whole plum tomatoes in your hands to break them up or quickly whizz them in a food processor. Stir in the grated garlic and tomato purée and season generously with salt and pepper.

Make the pizza dough (see opposite). Top each pizza base with a fairly thin layer of marinara sauce – 2–3 tablespoons willl be enough. Sprinkle with a few slices of garlic, cherry tomato halves and a pinch of dried oregano, if you like.

Cook the pizzas as instructed above. Enjoy hot with a drizzle of olive oil.

PIZZA CAPONATA

SERVES 3-4

3 tablespoons olive oil, plus
   extra for drizzling
1 small aubergine, cut into
   small cubes
1 quantity Homemade Pizza
   Dough (see page 88)
1 quantity Marinara Sauce
   (see page 89)
15-20 black or green olives,
   halved
3-4 tablespoons drained
   capers
½ red onion, finely sliced
small handful of basil leaves
   (optional)
Vegan Parmesan (see page
   120, optional)

Sharp and sweet, caponata deserves to be much more than a dip. Think of this as the vegan equivalent of an anchovy and olive number. (See photo on page 86.)

Heat the olive oil in a large frying pan and sauté the aubergine until tender and golden brown.

Make the pizza dough (see pages 88-9). Top each pizza base with a few tablespoons of marinara sauce, a handful of aubergine pieces, 5 olives, 1 tablespoon of capers and a few red onion slices.

Cook the pizzas as instructed on page 89. Enjoy hot with a drizzle of olive oil, with some basil and vegan parmesan, if you like.

COURGETTE, LEMON & MINT PIZZA

SERVES 3-4

1 quantity Homemade Pizza
   Dough (see page 88)
½ quantity Breadcrumb Pesto
   (see page 70)
1 courgette, finely sliced
1 red chilli, finely sliced,
   deseeded if you prefer
   less heat
extra virgin olive oil or
   regular olive oil, for
   drizzling
finely grated zest of 1 lemon
small handful of mint leaves
Vegan Parmesan (see page
   120, optional)

Incredibly fresh, this will help use up any Breadcrumb Pesto (see page 70) and makes a nice change to a tomato-based pizza topping. (See photo on page 86.)

Make the pizza dough (see pages 88-9). Top each pizza base with a few tablespoons of breadcrumb pesto, followed by a large handful of courgette and some red chilli slices.

Cook the pizzas as instructed on page 89. Enjoy hot with a drizzle of olive oil and a scattering of lemon zest and mint leaves, with vegan parmesan, if you like.

MUSHROOM, SPINACH & GARLIC PIZZA

SERVES 3–4

100 g (3½ oz) unsalted cashew
    nuts, soaked in cold water
    overnight, or soaked in
    boiling water for 1 hour
3 tablespoons lemon juice
2 tablespoons extra virgin olive
    oil or regular olive oil, plus
    extra for drizzling
300 g (10 oz) mushrooms,
    finely sliced
200 g (7 oz) spinach
1 quantity Homemade Pizza
    Dough (see page 88)
2 garlic cloves, finely sliced
Vegan Parmesan (see page
    120, optional)
salt and pepper

The cashew cream base in this recipe mimics a traditional white-based pizza bianca, which has no tomato sauce. Don't be afraid to add lots of lemon juice: it is needed to bring the toppings to life.

Drain and rinse the soaked cashews and blitz in a food processor with the lemon juice and a few splashes of water until you have a very smooth and creamy sauce, just thicker than double cream. Season to taste.

Heat the olive oil in a large frying pan and sauté the mushrooms until tender and golden brown (this will take 5–6 minutes). Turn off the heat, add the spinach to the pan and allow to wilt.

Make the pizza dough (see pages 88–9). Top each pizza base with a few tablespoons of cashew cream, followed by a large handful of mushrooms and spinach and some garlic slices.

Cook the pizzas as instructed on page 89. Enjoy hot with a drizzle of olive oil and vegan parmesan, if you like.

PESTO & CONFIT TOMATO PIZZA

SERVES 3–4

1 quantity Homemade Pizza
    Dough (see page 88)
½ quantity Breadcrumb Pesto
    (see page 70)
250 g (8 oz) Confit Tomatoes
    (see page 38)
extra virgin olive oil or regular
    olive oil, for drizzling
large handful of basil leaves
Vegan Parmesan (see page
    120)

If you've been organized about batch cooking, this pizza should be able to be topped with things you already have in your cupboard and refrigerator, and it will be your guests' favourite, guaranteed.

Make the pizza dough (see pages 88–9). Top each pizza base with a few tablespoons of breadcrumb pesto, followed by a large handful of confit tomatoes.

Cook the pizzas as instructed on page 89. Enjoy hot with a drizzle of olive oil and a sprinkling of basil leaves and vegan parmesan.

HOMEMADE PASTA

Making your own pasta couldn't be easier or cheaper. You only need two ingredients: flour and water. And it's wonderful pre-dinner entertainment for your guests too – get them rolling out your shape of choice and everyone will be that bit more invested in their meal. Using semolina flour here really does make all the difference to the texture, but you can use plain flour or strong white bread flour if you must and no one would be the wiser.

SERVES 6

600 g (1 lb 5 oz) semolina flour, plus extra for dusting
1½ teaspoons fine salt
575 ml (18 fl oz) warm water
sauce of your choice (see pages 95–7)

Put the semolina flour and salt on a clean work top and make a well in the middle. Gradually add the measured water, using your hand or a wooden spoon to work it into the flour gradually. It will seem very dry at first, but keep kneading and bringing it together until it is a cohesive mass. You should not need to add any more water, as you don't want the dough to become sticky, so make sure you have weighed and measured everything correctly. Knead it for 8–10 minutes until it is smooth and soft to the touch.

Wrap the dough in clingfilm and rest at room temperature for at least 30 minutes and up to 5 hours.

Once the dough has rested, sprinkle a baking tray with semolina flour. Form the dough into the desired shapes, depending on which type of pasta you have chosen (see page 94), and place them on the semolina-dusted baking tray to prevent any sticking.

Once you've made your sauce (see pages 95–7), bring a large saucepan of water to the boil with plenty of salt and cook the pasta until al dente (this will take 6–8 minutes). Drain the pasta, reserving some of the cooking water to add to the sauce, if needed.

If not cooking the pasta straight away, cover the tray and leave in the refrigerator for up to 2 days. Or freeze the shapes spaced apart on the tray, then transfer to an airtight container where they'll keep for 2 months and can be cooked from frozen – just add 1 minute to the cooking time.

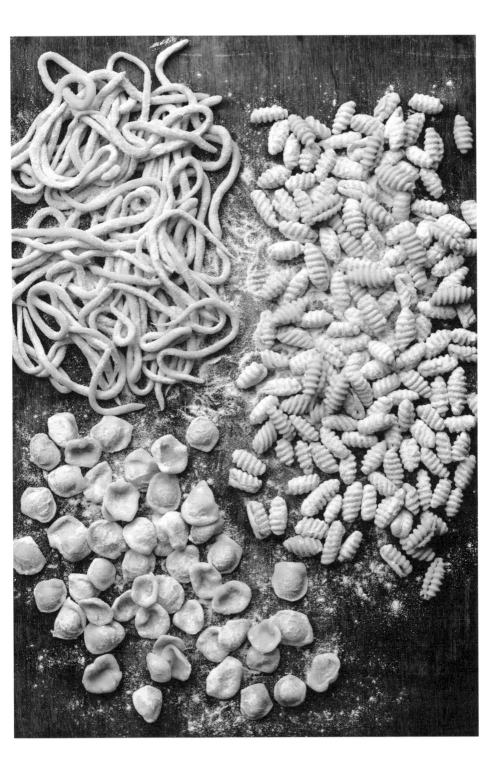

CAVATELLI

After the dough has rested, and keeping the bulk of it covered, pinch off a golf ball-sized piece of dough. Roll it into a long log around 1 cm (½ inch) in diameter. Use a knife or bench scraper to cut the log into 2.5 cm (1 inch) pieces.

Using your fingers and firm pressure, roll the piece of dough along a ridged paddle, or a fork, until the pasta curls in on itself and leaves a hollow crevice in the centre. Alternatively you can just use your index and middle finger to press on the piece of dough, curling it towards you to create a ridgeless cavatelli.

Repeat with the rest of the dough.

ORECCHIETTE

After the dough has rested, and keeping the bulk of it covered, pinch off a golf ball-sized piece of dough. Roll it into a long log around 1 cm (½ inch) in diameter. Use a knife or bench scraper to cut the log into 2.5 cm (1 inch) pieces.

Using the flat tip of a table knife at a 45-degree angle, with 2 fingers on the flat side for pressure, drag the piece of dough towards you, then use your thumb to invert the shape, making it look a bit like an ear.

Repeat with the rest of the dough.

PICI

After the dough has rested, and keeping the bulk of it covered, pinch off a golf ball-sized piece of dough. Roll it into a long log around 1 cm (½ inch) in diameter. Use a knife or bench scraper to cut the log into 2.5 cm (1 inch) pieces.

Roll each piece into a long even rope, like a piece of spaghetti but longer and thicker, tapering somewhat at the ends.

Repeat with the rest of the dough.

BUTTERNUT SQUASH & SAGE PICI

SERVES 6

1 large butternut squash,
    peeled and cut into 2.5 cm
    (1 inch) cubes
5 tablespoons extra virgin
    olive oil or regular olive oil
1 shallot, quartered
2 garlic cloves, in their skins
300–400 ml (½ pint–14 fl oz)
    vegan stock
¼ teaspoon freshly grated
    nutmeg
1 tablespoon sherry vinegar
    or red wine vinegar
1 quantity Pici pasta (see
    pages 92–4)
handful of sage leaves
salt and pepper

*This smooth, vibrant orange sauce is sweet, sharp and
completely addictive slathered over the delightfully chewy pici.*

Preheat the oven to 180°C (350°F), Gas Mark 4.

Put the squash on a baking tray and toss in 3 tablespoons of
the oil. Season and roast for 20 minutes. Add the shallot and
garlic and roast for 10–15 minutes until the squash is tender.

Squeeze the garlic out of their skins and transfer to a blender
with the shallots and three-quarters of the squash. Add the
stock and blitz. Season with nutmeg, vinegar, salt and pepper.

Cook the pici as instructed on page 92.

Meanwhile, heat the remaining oil in a large saucepan and fry
the sage leaves for 1 minute until crisp, then remove them and
drain on kitchen paper.

When cooked, spoon the pasta directly into the pan with the
sage oil. Add the squash sauce and toss to combine, ladling in
a splash of the pasta cooking water to loosen the sauce. Divide
the pici between warmed serving bowls and top with the
reserved butternut squash pieces and the crispy sage.

CLASSIC POMODORO CAVATELLI

SERVES 6

4 tablespoons extra virgin
    olive oil or regular olive oil,
    plus extra for drizzling
5 garlic cloves, finely
    chopped or grated
2 x 400 g (13 oz) cans plum
    tomatoes
1 teaspoon caster sugar
1 tablespoon balsamic
    vinegar
1 quantity Cavatelli pasta
    (see pages 92–4)
salt and pepper

*Spaghetti with tomato sauce is the ultimate cheap meal, but
when you make your own pasta you elevate it to the next
level. Add sugar and balsamic vinegar to taste.*

Heat the oil in a heavy-based frying pan. Add the garlic and
cook for 1–2 minutes. Add the plum tomatoes, squashing them
to break them up. Fill a tomato can with water and add to the
pan. Add the sugar and a pinch of salt and cook over a low
heat for 1 hour until reduced and thickened significantly. Add
the balsamic vinegar and season to taste. Turn off the heat.

Cook the cavatelli as instructed on page 92. Reheat the
tomato sauce if necessary, then spoon the pasta directly
into the sauce and toss to combine, ladling in a splash of the
pasta cooking water to loosen the sauce. Serve with an extra
grinding of pepper and a drizzle of olive oil.

BROCCOLI, GARLIC, LEMON & CHILLI ORECCHIETTE

SERVES 6

1 large head of broccoli,
broken into florets, stem
roughly chopped
1 quantity Orecchiette pasta
(see pages 92–4)
50 ml (2 fl oz) extra virgin
olive oil or regular olive oil
4 garlic cloves, finely sliced
finely grated zest and juice
of 1 lemon
2 teaspoons chilli flakes
3 tablespoons Vegan
Parmesan (see page 120)
salt and pepper

This is a delicious broccoli sauce, but if you only have the garlic, chilli and lemon, that's also a banging budget supper.

Bring a large saucepan of salted water to the boil. Add the broccoli and blanch for 3 minutes until just tender. Transfer to a chopping board and allow the broccoli to cool briefly, then roughly chop it into smaller bite-sized pieces.

Cook the orecchiette as instructed on page 92.

Meanwhile, heat the oil in a large frying pan over a medium heat. Add the garlic and fry for 1–2 minutes until fragrant and lightly golden.

Add the cooked pasta to the frying pan with the broccoli. Season with the lemon zest and juice and add the chilli flakes. Toss everything together vigorously until the starch releases from the pasta to thicken the sauce, adding a splash of pasta water if necessary to loosen it. Serve with the vegan parmesan and a generous amount of pepper.

PICI WITH CHERRY TOMATOES, SPINACH & COURGETTES

SERVES 6

25 cherry tomatoes
2 courgettes, sliced
2 garlic cloves, finely
chopped or grated
3 tablespoons extra virgin
olive oil or regular olive oil,
plus extra for drizzling
1 quantity Pici pasta (see
pages 92–4)
350 g (11½ oz) spinach
3 tablespoons Vegan
Parmesan (see page 120),
plus extra to serve
salt and pepper

This fresh and summery pasta dish makes the most of seasonal produce. Replace the cherry tomatoes with Confit Tomatoes (see page 38), if you like.

Preheat the oven to 180°C (350°F), Gas Mark 4.

Toss the tomatoes, courgettes and garlic with 2 tablespoons of the oil in a baking tray. Roast for 30 minutes until tender and beginning to colour.

Cook the pici as instructed on page 92.

Return the pici to the saucepan with the remaining olive oil and add the roasted cherry tomatoes and courgettes. Add the spinach and a splash of the pasta cooking water and toss vigorously to combine. Serve with vegan parmesan, a generous amount of pepper and a drizzle of olive oil.

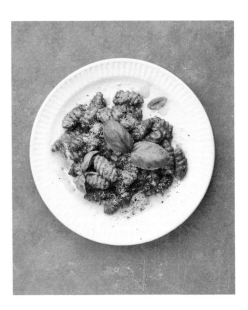

CAVOLO NERO CAVATELLI

SERVES 6

500 g (1 lb) cavolo nero, kale
    or spinach
3 garlic cloves
1 quantity Cavatelli pasta
    (see pages 92–4)
3 tablespoons extra virgin
    olive oil or regular olive oil,
    plus extra to serve
3 tablespoons Vegan
    Parmesan (see page 120),
    plus extra to serve
small handful of basil leaves
    (optional)
salt

This works with any leafy greens – try rocket, spring greens or green cabbage.

Bring a large saucepan of salted water to the boil. Add the cavolo nero and garlic cloves and blanch for 3 minutes. Remove with a slotted spoon and run under cold water to stop the cooking, then transfer to a blender.

Using the same salted water, cook the cavatelli as instructed on page 92.

Take a cupful or two of pasta water and add to the blender along with the oil and vegan parmesan, then blitz until you have a smooth and vibrant green sauce.

Toss the cavatelli with the green sauce in the large saucepan, adding more pasta water if the sauce seems too thick. Serve with a sprinkling of vegan parmesan and basil leaves, if using.

TACO NIGHT TORTILLAS

These tortillas can be cooked ahead of time and reheated when you need them. You can try baking them moulded over an upturned muffin tray to make little bowls or they're wonderful deep-fried as tostadas. Masa harina is ground maize flour and is not expensive at all, but you can swap it for plain flour if you can't find any.

MAKES 12–16

200 g (7 oz) masa harina,
   plus extra for dusting or
   as needed
¼ teaspoon salt
2 tablespoons vegetable oil
175 ml (6 fl oz) hot water,
   plus extra if needed

Combine the masa harina and salt in a large bowl and add the oil. Pour in the measured water in a steady stream and mix everything together with your hands.

Knead the dough in the bowl for 5–8 minutes until it feels smooth but firm. Masa is gluten-free, so it won't knead like a traditional bread dough – if it seems too dry and crumbly, add a little more hot water, or if it is too wet add more flour.

Wrap tightly in clingfilm and allow to rest at room temperature for at least 30 minutes and up to 5 hours.

Divide the dough into 12–16 pieces, depending on the size you'd like, and roll each piece into a ball. Choose 1 ball (cover the rest) and place it between the 2 sheets of a split freezer bag (this works better than clingfilm, which is a bit wrinkly) or nonstick baking paper. Roll out with a rolling pin, or use a heavy-based saucepan or casserole dish to push the ball out into a thin circle. (If the tortilla doesn't roll off the plastic easily it's probably too wet. Add a little extra flour and rest again for 30 minutes.)

Cook the tortilla in a hot, dry frying pan for 1–2 minutes on each side until brown spots start to appear.

Shape and fry the remaining tortillas, one at a time. (Because they are gluten-free, they need to go straight from being pressed into the pan or they will be hard to handle.) Keep them warm, wrapped in a tea towel, until they are all ready to serve. Store, wrapped in clingfilm, at room temperature for up to 2 days.

BLACK BEAN TACOS

SERVES 6

Salsa (optional)
125 g (4 oz) pomegranate
  seeds
1 green chilli, deseeded and
  finely chopped
½ red onion, finely chopped
small handful of coriander,
  finely chopped, plus extra
  to serve

1 quantity Whole-can Tangy
  Black Beans (see page 37)
1 quantity Taco Night Tortillas
  (see opposite)
1 lime, cut into wedges, to
  serve

A quick pomegranate salsa adds freshness and crunch to these tacos, but in all honesty you can do without it – just piling the tangy black beans on fresh tortillas with a little coriander is plenty delicious enough.

To make the salsa, if using, mix together all the ingredients.

Reheat the black beans. Spread them over the tortillas, topping with the pomegranate salsa, if using.

Serve with coriander and lime wedges.

CAULIFLOWER AL PASTOR TACOS

SERVES 6

1 avocado, halved, peeled,
  pitted and sliced
1 quantity Taco Night Tortillas
  (see opposite)
1 quantity Cauliflower
  Nuggets (see page 79)
1 quantity Pineapple Salsa
  (see page 114)

To serve
small handful of coriander,
  roughly chopped
1 lime, cut into wedges
hot sauce

For an extra smoky dimension to these sweet and crunchy tacos, try grilling the pineapple before adding it to the salsa.

Lay 2 slices of avocado on each tortilla and top with the cauliflower nuggets and pineapple salsa.

Serve with coriander, lime wedges and hot sauce.

SMOKY MUSHROOM TACO BOWLS

SERVES 6

3 tablespoons flavourless oil,
   plus extra for oiling
1 quantity Taco Night Tortillas
   (see page 98)
500 g (1 lb) chestnut
   mushrooms, finely sliced
2 garlic cloves, grated
2 teaspoons smoked paprika
2 tablespoons tomato purée
1 quantity Limey Cashew
   Cream (see page 46)
5 radishes, finely sliced
½ onion, finely chopped
coriander sprigs

Use any mushroom you can find to make these little taco bowls – oyster mushrooms are particularly good. The tacos are twice cooked so are a good way to use up any leftover tortillas.

Preheat the oven to 180°C (350°F), Gas Mark 4. Oil the underside of a muffin tray, place a tortilla around each mould, then bake for 10 minutes until crisp and holding their bowl shapes. Set aside.

Heat the oil in a large frying pan. Add the mushrooms and cook for 5–6 minutes until golden brown. Add the garlic and cook for a further minute, followed by the paprika and tomato purée. Add a splash of water and cook for a further 2 minutes.

Fill each taco bowl with a few tablespoons of smoky mushrooms and a dollop of limey cashew cream. Garnish with radishes, onion and coriander.

CHARGRILLED CORN & PEPPER TACOS

SERVES 6

2 x 300 g (10 oz) cans
   sweetcorn, drained
2 red peppers, cored,
   deseeded and finely sliced
2 green peppers, cored,
   deseeded and finely sliced
1 tablespoon ground cumin
finely grated zest and juice
   of 1 lime
1 quantity Taco Night Tortillas
   (see page 98)
salt and pepper

To serve
1 quantity Tomato Salsa
   (see page 114)
coriander sprigs

Try chargrilling any vegetables that you'd like here – courgette, aubergine or cabbage all work really well. (See photo opposite.)

Preheat a large dry frying pan over a high heat. Add the sweetcorn and peppers and cook for 6–7 minutes until charred and blistered. Take off the heat and sprinkle with the cumin, lime zest and juice. Season with salt and pepper.

Serve the vegetables in the tacos with tomato salsa and coriander.

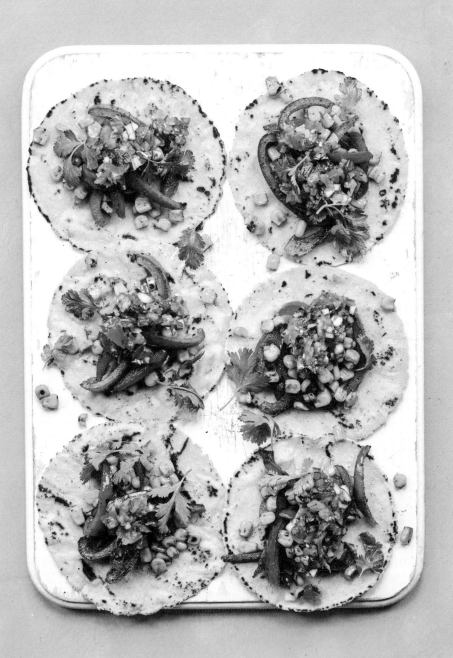

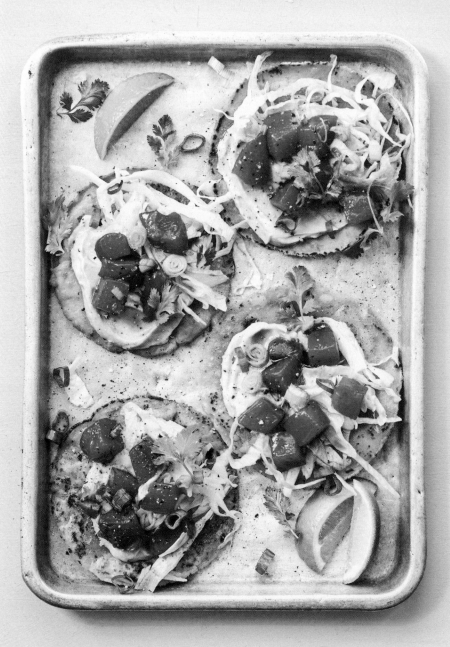

SPICY 'TUNA' WATERMELON TOSTADAS

Roasting watermelon concentrates its flavour and lends it a firmer texture. Any leftovers of this spicy-sweet topping are also great served on a vegan poke bowl or just eaten with rice.

SERVES 6

1 small watermelon (about
    1.25 kg / 2½ lb), peeled
3 tablespoons soy sauce
finely grated zest and juice
    of 1 lime
2 tablespoons finely chopped
    pickled jalapeños
2 tablespoons sriracha or
    other hot sauce
flavourless oil, to deep-fry
1 quantity Taco Night Tortillas
    (see page 98)
salt

To serve
1 quantity Avocado Crema
    (optional, see page 114)
shredded lettuce
spring onions, finely sliced
small handful of coriander,
    roughly chopped
1 lime, cut into wedges

Preheat the oven to 200°C (400°F), Gas Mark 6. Roast the watermelon on a large baking tray for 2 hours until shrunken slightly, charred and softened. Leave to cool, then slice, cube and transfer to a bowl with any roasting juices from the baking tray.

Add the soy sauce, lime zest and juice, pickled jalapeños and hot sauce to the bowl and leave to marinate for 1 hour.

Heat 1 cm (½ inch) of oil in a large frying pan. Fry the tortillas for 1 minute on each side until crisp and golden. Drain on kitchen paper and season with salt.

Top each tostada with the spicy watermelon cubes, avocado crema, if using, shredded lettuce, spring onions, coriander and lime wedges.

ANY VEGETABLE TART 101

A tart is an art, but is such an easy crowd-pleaser. It can mostly be cooked ahead of time, or at least prepared and refrigerated before your guests come over. Follow these basic rules and you'll have success every time. It goes without saying to make sure that all the pastry you buy is vegan, but luckily this is standard in most supermarkets.

CHOOSE YOUR PASTRY & TREAT IT RIGHT

SHORTCRUST PASTRY

These pastry cases need to be blind-baked before filling. To do this, preheat the oven to 180°C (350°F), Gas Mark 4. Roll the pastry out to fit the chosen tin, prick it with a fork all over, then chill. Line the pastry case with a piece of nonstick baking paper and fill with baking beans or raw rice or dried beans. Bake for 15 minutes, until the pastry is sandy to the touch with no uncooked patches. Remove the baking paper and cook for a further 5 minutes until lightly golden, before adding your chosen filling.

It's easier to trim off any overhanging pastry after blind-baking and this also helps avoid the pastry shrinking during cooking. Use a serrated knife to trim the pastry edges while still warm.

PUFF PASTRY

Puff pastry doesn't need to be blind-baked. If making a puff pastry tart, roll it out and score 2 cm (1 inch) around the edge. Prick the centre of the pastry with a fork to help the edges puff up and the base to cook without becoming soggy.

Preheat a baking tray while you preheat the oven to 190°C (375°F), Gas Mark 5. Sliding a puff pastry tart on to a hot baking sheet will give an instant hit of heat from below, so no soggy bottoms.

Brush the pastry with 1 tablespoon or so of dairy-free milk on any exposed edges to help it to brown evenly.

FILO PASTRY

Brush this with a little bit of oil between every layer to ensure you get flaky shards. Filo doesn't need to be blind-baked, but when it's in the oven you may sometimes need to cover it with foil to prevent it from browning too quickly.

It's quite show-stopping if you scrunch up filo pastry to top a pie filling, or you can use it to make spanakopita-style swirls.

CHOOSE YOUR SHAPE & SIZE

Tarts are wonderful served individually. This works pretty well for puff pastry tarts, which don't require any special tins and can just be baked straight on a baking tray.

Try using an ovenproof frying pan for filo pastry tarts, for quick weeknight suppers, if you don't have a tart tin.

If you don't have a circular or fluted tart tin, use a deep baking tray for shortcrust pastry tarts.

FLAVOURS & TEXTURES

Almost every successful tart balances texture and flavour contrasts. Use the following formula for foolproof tart combinations:

Use a thick sauce or spread – think pesto, super-caramelized onions, puréed butternut squash or hummus. This will help your vegetables to stay in place and act as a barrier between them and the pastry.

Consider pre-cooking vegetables. Sometimes twice-cooked vegetables are the key to a tart's success, especially if you're using vegetables that release a lot of moisture, such as tomatoes or courgettes.

ADDED EXTRAS

Whether it's a sprinkling of lemon zest and capers, hot sauce or Crispy Chickpeas (see page 121), think what's going to be nice to look at when the tart comes out of the oven – little bonuses drizzled or sprinkled on top make everything more appetizing.

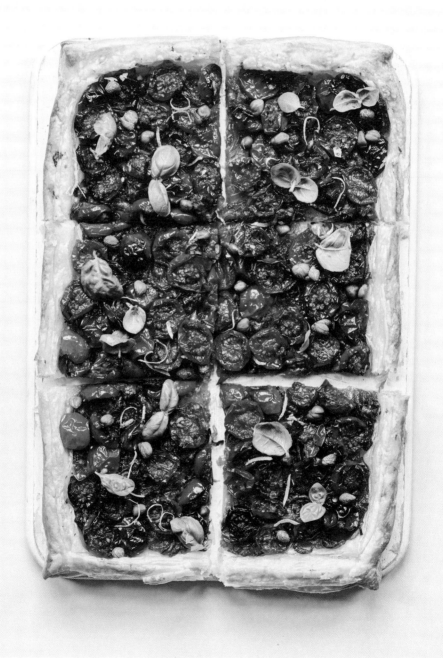

CARAMELIZED SHALLOT & TOMATO TART

You need to caramelize the shallots thoroughly here to unleash their flavour – it takes a while, but if you cook double you can use the leftovers in other tarts, in a quesadilla (see page 76) or use them as a base for a quick soup.

SERVES 4-6

1 quantity Confit Tomatoes
   (see page 38)
6 shallots, finely sliced
1 teaspoon caster sugar
1 tablespoon red wine
   vinegar
200 g (7 oz) block vegan
   puff pastry
1 tablespoon dairy-free milk
   (optional)
3 tablespoons drained capers
finely grated zest of 1 lemon
leaves from 3 basil sprigs

Preheat the oven to 190°C (375°F), Gas Mark 5. Place a baking sheet or large baking tray in the oven to heat up.

Use 3 tablespoons of the oil from the confit tomatoes to fry the shallots in a large frying pan over a medium heat for 10 minutes until softened. Add the sugar and red wine vinegar and cook for a further 10 minutes until sticky and caramelized.

Roll the puff pastry out into a rectangle on a large sheet of nonstick baking paper and score a smaller rectangle 2.5 cm (1 inch) from the edge. Prick the inner rectangle with a fork, then cover with a layer of caramelized shallots.

Top evenly with the drained confit tomatoes. Brush the exposed edges of the pastry with the milk, if you like, slide the tart on its paper onto the preheated baking sheet or tray and bake for 25–30 minutes until the pastry is golden. Sprinkle the tart with the capers, lemon zest and basil leaves to serve.

SPINACH, PEA & MINT FILO TART

This tart has spanakopita vibes and brings a taste of spring right to your table.

SERVES 6

2 tablespoons olive oil, plus extra for brushing the pastry

300 g (10 oz) frozen peas, defrosted

300 g (10 oz) frozen spinach, defrosted and squeezed of all excess water

5 spring onions, finely sliced

1 quantity Pea & Mint Pesto (see page 71)

½ teaspoon freshly grated nutmeg

320 g (11 oz) packet vegan filo pastry sheets

leaves from 3 mint sprigs

finely grated zest of 1 lemon

salt and pepper

Preheat the oven to 200°C (400°F), Gas Mark 6.

Heat the oil in a large frying pan and fry the peas, spinach and spring onions with a pinch of salt over a medium heat until no liquid remains in the pan and the spring onions are soft.

Turn off the heat and stir in the pesto, then season with nutmeg, salt and pepper.

Layer the filo sheets in a large deep baking tin, overlapping each sheet, and brushing each layer with olive oil, until the whole tin (and its sides) is lined with filo.

Spread the filling evenly across the middle, then scrunch up the overhanging pastry to form an edge.

Bake for 15 minutes until the filling is firm and the pastry is deep golden brown. Sprinkle with the mint leaves and lemon zest and serve.

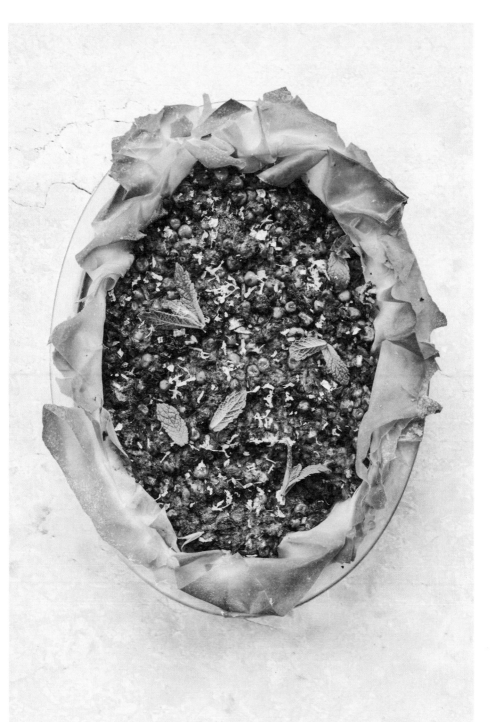

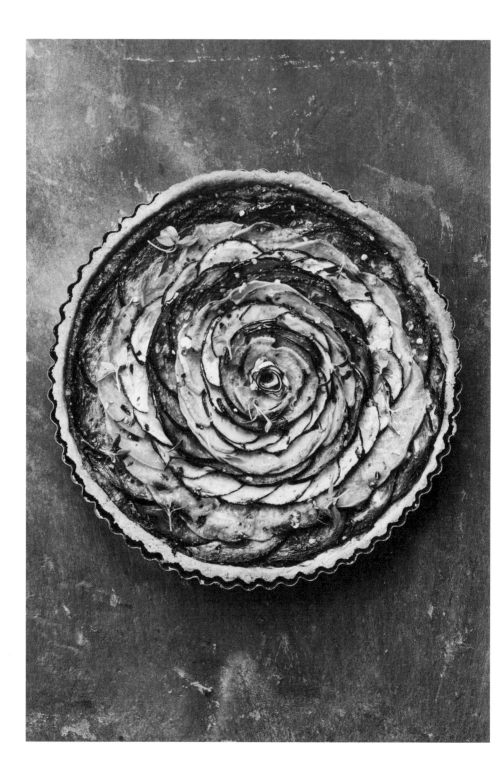

SPIRAL TART

This finely sliced vegetable tart is a total show-stopper and all it requires is a little bit of your time to decorate it.

SERVES 6

500 g (1 lb) block vegan
    shortcrust pastry
plain flour, for dusting
1–2 courgettes
1–2 sweet potatoes, peeled
1 aubergine
2 garlic cloves, crushed
2 tablespoons olive oil
1 quantity Breadcrumb Pesto
    (see page 70)
leaves from 3 thyme sprigs
1 tablespoon chilli flakes
salt and pepper

Preheat the oven to 180°C (350°F), Gas Mark 4.

Roll out the shortcrust pastry on a lightly floured work top to 1.5 cm (¾ inch) thick and use it to line a 25 cm (10 inch) fluted tart tin. Prick the base with a fork and blind bake (see page 104).

Meanwhile, trim the ends off the vegetables, slice them thinly, then cut into half-moon shapes. Toss the vegetables with the garlic and oil in a large bowl.

Spread the pesto over the base of the pastry case. To decorate, place a circle of aubergine half moons around the edge of the tart, then a circle of sweet potato, then a circle of courgette, alternating the vegetables until the base is filled, to create a flower-like pattern.

Sprinkle with thyme and chilli flakes, season well with salt and pepper, then bake for 40 minutes until the vegetables are tender and cooked through. Check after 20 minutes and cover the edges of the pastry with foil if they seem to be catching during the long cooking time.

BEETROOT TARTE TATIN

SERVES 6

320 g (11 oz) block vegan
   puff pastry
2 tablespoons olive oil
2 red onions, finely sliced
1 tablespoon caster sugar
1 tablespoon balsamic
   vinegar
leaves from 2 thyme sprigs,
   plus extra to serve
400 g (13 oz) cooked
   beetroot, cut into wedges
salt and pepper

This uses vacuum-packed beetroots that are readily available in supermarkets (just make sure they're not pickled in vinegar).

Preheat the oven to 200°C (400°F), Gas Mark 6.

Roll out the pastry to 5 mm (¼ inch) thick. Use a dinner plate as large as the ovenproof frying pan in which you will cook the tarte, as a template to cut out a circle of pastry and place on some nonstick baking paper. Transfer this to a tray and keep in the refrigerator until you need it.

Heat the oil in the ovenproof frying pan and fry the red onions for 15 minutes over a low heat or until deeply caramelized. Sprinkle over the sugar, vinegar and thyme and stir well to combine. Add the beetroot wedges in a snug single layer in a concentric circle pattern. Turn off the heat.

Cover the onions and beetroots with the puff pastry circle, tucking the edges down the side of the pan.

Bake for 30 minutes until the pastry is golden and well risen. Remove from the oven and leave to stand for 10 minutes before inverting onto a large serving dish. Scatter with thyme leaves and season well with salt and pepper.

MINI HUMMUS & CARROT TARTS

MAKES 4

320 g (11 oz) sheet ready-
   rolled vegan puff pastry
1 tablespoon dairy-free milk
1 quantity Any Can Hummus
   (see page 115)
1 quantity Maple Roast
   Carrots (see page 28)
50 g (2 oz) green olives,
   pitted and halved
50 g (2 oz) pomegranate
   seeds (optional)
large handful of flat leaf
   parsley, finely chopped

You can swap the hummus for pesto or use any roasted vegetables instead of the carrots.

Preheat the oven to 190°C (375°F), Gas Mark 5.

Cut the sheet of puff pastry into 4 rectangles and place on a large baking tray. Score a 2.5 cm (1 inch) border around each edge and prick the centres with a fork. Brush the outer edges with the milk. Bake for 12–15 minutes until risen and golden. Remove from the oven and push down the centre rectangles with the back of a spoon.

Spread the hummus in the centre of each tart, top with the carrots and olives and return to the oven for 5 minutes to warm through. Scatter the tarts with the pomegranate seeds, if using, and parsley before serving.

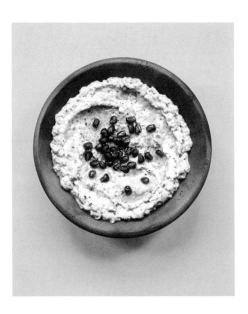

BABA GHANOUSH

Smoky and sharp, this dip is wonderful on its own or as a base for
a chopped salad with cucumber, tomato and red onion. It's a great
way to use up any forgotten-about wrinkly aubergines.

SERVES 6 AS AN
ACCOMPANIMENT

2 aubergines
1 garlic clove, grated
2 tablespoons tahini
2 tablespoons lemon juice
1 tablespoon extra virgin olive
    oil or regular olive oil, plus
    extra to serve
1 teaspoon maple syrup
pomegranate seeds, to serve
    (optional)
salt and pepper

If you have a gas hob, place the aubergines directly over
the flame and cook for 15–20 minutes, turning using tongs,
until completely blistered and blackened and soft inside.
(Alternatively, you can do this under the grill.)

Halve the aubergines and scoop out the flesh, discarding
the blackened skins.

Finely chop the aubergine flesh and transfer to a bowl.
Mix with the garlic, tahini, lemon juice, oil and maple syrup
and season to taste. Top with a drizzle of olive oil to serve,
adding pomegranate seeds, if you like.

This will keep in an airtight container in the refrigerator for
up to 4 days.

5 DIPS & SALSAS

ALL SERVE 6 AS AN ACCOMPANIMENT

AVOCADO CREMA

2 avocados, halved, peeled
   and pitted
3 tablespoons lime juice
salt and pepper

Avocados have a bad 'expensive' reputation, but this easy dip makes an over- or under-ripe avocado into something delicious, and you only need a little to add a spot of luxury to your food.

Put the avocados and lime juice into a blender and blitz until smooth, adding 1 tablespoon of water if needed. Season well.

Store with a strip of clingfilm pushed firmly and directly on the surface of the dip, to prevent it from browning.

TOMATO SALSA

1 red onion, finely chopped
400 g (13 oz) tomatoes,
   roughly chopped
1 garlic clove, grated
large handful of coriander,
   finely chopped
finely grated zest and juice
   of 2 limes
1 red chilli, deseeded and
   finely chopped (optional)
salt and pepper

It's up to you whether you want this to be spicy or not, so feel free to leave out the chilli if you want something more neutral. This is wonderful served with Sweet Potato Quesadillas or tacos (see pages 76 and 98–100).

Mix all the ingredients together and season to taste.

PINEAPPLE SALSA

1 small pineapple, chopped
   into 1 cm (½ inch) cubes
1 small red onion, finely
   chopped
1 red chilli, deseeded and
   finely chopped
small handful of coriander,
   finely chopped
finely grated zest and juice
   of 2 limes
salt and pepper

Serve this with Chilli Con Veggie, Sweet Potato Quesadillas or tacos (see pages 48, 76 and 98–100). Canned pineapple, drained and rinsed, works just as well as fresh pineapple. You can also substitute the pineapple for mango or watermelon, if you prefer.

Mix all the ingredients together and season to taste.

ANY CAN HUMMUS

400 g (13 oz) can chickpeas
  or any other canned bean
¼ teaspoon bicarbonate of
  soda
4 tablespoons tahini
2–3 tablespoons lemon juice
1 teaspoon ground cumin
1 garlic clove, grated
salt and pepper

To serve (optional)
extra virgin olive oil or
  regular olive oil
chilli flakes

The trick to smooth hummus is to recook the canned beans with bicarbonate of soda until they are incredibly tender. No need for the traditional and very laborious peeling of the chickpea skins, yet no grainy dips in sight – life changing.

Put the chickpeas, or other beans, and their liquid into a small saucepan with the bicarbonate of soda. Bring to the boil, then reduce the heat to a simmer and cook for 15 minutes until extremely tender.

Drain the chickpeas, reserving the liquid.

Blitz the chickpeas with the tahini, 2 tablespoons of the lemon juice, the cumin and garlic until smooth, adding 4–5 tablespoons of the reserved liquid from the saucepan, until incredibly smooth and creamy. Season to taste, adding the remaining lemon juice if you want it.

Serve, drizzled with olive oil and chilli flakes, if you like.

ROASTED RED PEPPER DIP

2 red peppers, halved, cored
  and deseeded
2 large tomatoes, halved
3 tablespoons olive oil
1 tablespoon sherry vinegar
1 garlic clove, roughly
  chopped
1 teaspoon smoked paprika
150 g (5 oz) stale bread,
  ripped into pieces
salt and pepper

This is essentially a traditional Spanish Romesco sauce, but without the expensive almonds of the classic version. Try it with Charred Cauliflower Steaks (see page 116).

Preheat the oven to 220°C (425°F), Gas Mark 7.

Place the red peppers and tomatoes on a foil-lined baking tray, drizzle with 1 tablespoon of the oil, season and roast for 35 minutes until blistered, slightly charred and soft.

Remove and discard the skins from the peppers and tomatoes once they're cooked and add the rest to a blender with the remaining olive oil, the sherry vinegar, garlic, paprika and bread. Blitz until you have a rough and chunky dip. Season to taste and serve.

ROASTED CAULIFLOWER 5 WAYS

The humble cauliflower has had a surge in popularity in recent years, as people have discovered that – when treated correctly – it can be as satisfying a meal as any. Roasting cauliflower brings out all of the flavour. Only roast the leaves for the last 5–10 minutes; they taste like wonderful roasted kale. If you find a few florets come loose from their steaks, just chuck them on the tray to roast alongside.

CHARRED CAULIFLOWER STEAKS WITH HERBY GARLIC CRUMBS & ROASTED RED PEPPER DIP

SERVES 6

2 large cauliflowers, each sliced into 3 fat 'steaks' with the root attached

3 tablespoons extra virgin olive oil or regular olive oil

1 quantity Roasted Red Pepper Dip (see page 115)

1 quantity Chilli, Lemon & Herb Crumbs, with parsley (see page 121)

salt and pepper

These steaks look beautifully burnished on top of their vibrant orange dip. Perfect in the summertime, if you can cook the cauliflower on a barbecue.

Preheat the oven to 220°C (425°F), Gas Mark 7.

Lay the cauliflower steaks on a baking tray lined with nonstick baking paper. Coat well in the olive oil, being careful with the steaks as they can be quite delicate. Season well with salt and pepper and roast for 20–25 minutes, flipping halfway through and cooking until the steaks are charred and tender. Add the cauliflower leaves for the last 5–10 minutes.

Spread the red pepper dip on a large serving platter, top with the cauliflower steaks and sprinkle the flavoured crumbs over everything.

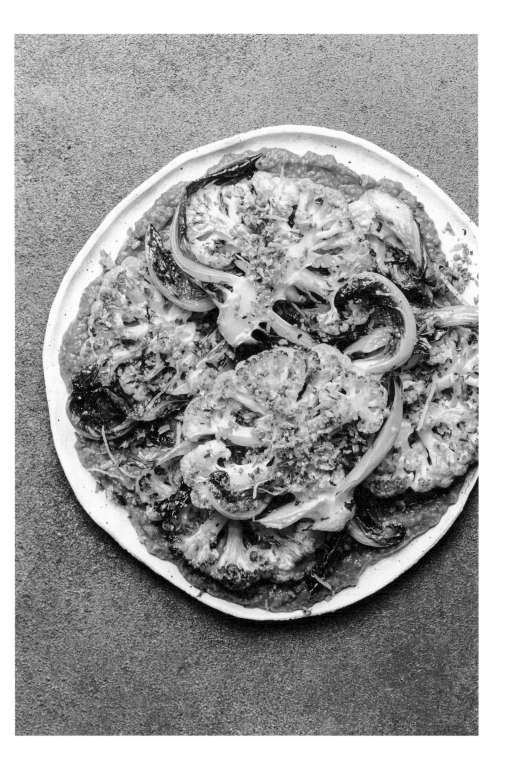

CAULIFLOWER STEAKS WITH OLIVES, CAPERS & OREGANO

SERVES 6

2 large cauliflowers, each sliced
    into 3 fat 'steaks' with the
    root attached
4 tablespoons olive oil
15 cherry tomatoes, halved
100 g (3½ oz) green olives,
    pitted and halved
100 g (3½ oz) drained capers
1 teaspoon dried oregano
large handful of flat leaf
    parsley, chopped, to serve

Sometimes it can be tricky to get good 'steaks' out of a cauliflower. But if all the florets fall apart and don't hold their shape, don't worry, just break the whole thing down and roast it as florets, adding the leaves for the last 10 minutes to crisp up.

Preheat the oven to 180°C (350°F), Gas Mark 4. Roast the cauliflower steaks with 3 tablespoons of the olive oil as on page 116, this time for 20 minutes.

Meanwhile, toss the cherry tomatoes, olives, capers and oregano with the remaining olive oil. After 20 minutes, flip the cauliflower steaks carefully and add the tomato mixture to the baking tray, taking care not to cover the cauliflower.

Cook for a further 20 minutes – adding the cauliflower leaves for the final 5–10 minutes – until the tomatoes are cooked and the cauliflower steak is charred and tender. Serve with a scattering of chopped parsley.

CAULIFLOWER STEAKS À LA FRANÇAISE

SERVES 6

2 large cauliflowers, each
    sliced into 3 fat 'steaks'
    with the root attached
4 tablespoons olive oil
3 spring onions, finely sliced
350 g (11½ oz) frozen peas
150 ml (¼ pint) vegan stock
1 Little Gem lettuce, finely
    shredded
finely grated zest and juice
    of 1 lemon
salt and pepper

Petits pois à la Française is a delicious side dish in which peas are braised with spring onions and lettuce. This cauliflower dish works perfectly with the same flavourings.

Preheat the oven to 180°C (350°F), Gas Mark 4. Bake the cauliflower steaks with 3 tablespoons of the olive oil as on page 116, this time for 30–35 minutes, adding the leaves for the final 5–10 minutes.

Meanwhile, add the remaining olive oil to a saucepan and cook the spring onions until soft. Add the peas and cook for 2 minutes before pouring in the stock. Allow the stock to boil up and mostly reduce away before stirring in the lettuce at the end so it just wilts. Season to taste and add the lemon zest and juice. Serve the cauliflower steaks on the bed of peas.

WHOLE MISO & HERB CAULIFLOWER

SERVES 6

2 large cauliflowers
2 tablespoons flavourless oil
large handful of coriander,
    finely chopped
salt and pepper

Marinade
2 tablespoons sesame oil
4 tablespoons miso paste
1 tablespoon caster sugar
finely grated zest and juice
    of 2 limes
1 tablespoon chilli flakes

This intensely savoury umami cauliflower will have any meat eaters around the table stunned. The recipe works well with any miso paste you have: white, red or brown.

Preheat the oven to 180°C (350°F), Gas Mark 4.

Rub the cauliflowers with the oil and season well. Roast whole for 25–30 minutes until almost tender.

Meanwhile, mix together all the ingredients for the marinade and set aside.

After 25–30 minutes, rub the cauliflowers with the marinade and cook for an additional 10–15 minutes until the marinade is sticky and sweet and the cauliflowers are completely tender.

Serve with a scattering of coriander.

WHOLE TIKKA CAULIFLOWER

SERVES 6

2 large cauliflowers
2 tablespoons flavourless oil
handful of coriander,
    chopped (optional)
salt and pepper

Marinade
200 ml (7 fl oz) can coconut
    milk
3 tablespoons tomato purée
1 teaspoon chilli powder
1 teaspoon garam masala
1 teaspoon ground cumin
1 teaspoon ground coriander
finely grated zest and juice
    of 1 lemon
3 garlic cloves, finely grated

You can leave out the ground spices and aromatics here and simply use a pot of vegan tikka curry paste mixed with the coconut milk and lemon zest to marinate the cauliflower if you prefer. Either way, to make it fancy, serve it with coriander.

Mix together half the coconut milk with all the other ingredients for the marinade and rub it all over the cauliflowers. Set aside for at least 1 hour to marinate.

Preheat the oven to 180°C (350°F), Gas Mark 4.

Season the cauliflowers well and drizzle the oil all over them. Roast on a baking tray for 40–45 minutes, with foil covering the top for the first 20 minutes to help the cauliflowers steam and cook through, before removing the foil so they can get caramelized and charred.

Serve with the remaining coconut milk, sprinkling with coriander, if you like.

5 CRISPY TOPPINGS

It's so important with vegan food that you don't forget about textural contrasts. An extra crunch can be the secret ingredient that makes your dish climb from good to great. Textural contrasts are very welcome on soft soups and stews, which are often some of the cheapest meals you can make. Try adding the garlic croutons to Spiced Squash Soup or topping dhal with the vegetable crisps (see pages 41 and 35). All these crispy toppings not only add crunch to any number of dishes, they also pack a flavourful punch.

VEGAN PARMESAN

FILLS A 200 G (7 OZ) JAR

75 g (3 oz) cashew nuts, peanuts or flaked almonds
3 tablespoons nutritional yeast
½ teaspoon salt

Store-bought 'vegan cheese' is expensive, stinks the refrigerator out and is mainly just processed coconut oil. This cheats' version blitzes nuts with nutritional yeast and salt. It keeps in a jar for months and livens up pizzas, pasta and tarts with its salty savouriness.

Whizz all the ingredients in a food processor until you have the texture of fine sand.

Pop in a jar and store at room temperature for up to 3 months.

GARLIC CROUTONS

SERVES 6

2 slices of stale bread, crusts cut off, torn into small pieces
2 tablespoons extra virgin olive oil or regular olive oil
1 garlic clove, grated
salt and pepper

When you've let your Cheat's Sourdough (see page 10) go stale, cut away the crusts and make a batch of these croutons, which keep in an airtight container for up to 2 weeks. If they get soft, just flash them back in the oven before serving.

Preheat the oven to 180°C (350°F), Gas Mark 4.

Toss the small pieces of bread in the olive oil and garlic on a baking sheet. Season well and bake for 15 minutes until golden brown.

CHILLI, LEMON & HERB CRUMBS

SERVES 6

50 ml (2 fl oz) olive oil
150 g (5 oz) breadcrumbs (or
    see recipe introduction)
1 tablespoon chilli flakes
finely grated zest of 1 lemon
1 tablespoon chopped herbs
    (try thyme, parsley or
    rosemary)

This can be made from stale bread whizzed up in a food processor – a delicious way to jazz up pasta and salads.

Heat the oil in a large frying pan and toss in the breadcrumbs. Fry for 3–4 minutes until golden and crisp.

Turn off the heat, then stir in the chilli flakes, lemon zest and herbs. Allow to cool, then store in an airtight container for up to 1 week.

CRISPY CHICKPEAS

SERVES 6

400 g (13 oz) can chickpeas,
    drained and rinsed
2 tablespoons extra virgin
    olive oil or regular olive oil
1 teaspoon spice of your
    choice (see recipe
    introduction)

The trick to these crispy chickpeas is to dry them thoroughly before baking. The spices make a real impact on the flavour – try smoked paprika, cumin, garam masala or ground coriander.

Preheat the oven to 190°C (375°F), Gas Mark 5.

Dry the chickpeas thoroughly, then toss with the olive oil and your chosen spice on a large baking sheet (they need lots of space around them to crisp up).

Bake for 20 minutes until crisp and golden.

VEGETABLE CRISPS

SERVES 6

300 g (10 oz) sweet potatoes,
    beetroots, carrots or
    parsnips, peeled
3 tablespoons olive oil
salt and pepper

Sweet potatoes, beetroots and parsnips all work well for this crispy topping. Try them on top of salads and risottos.

Preheat the oven to 180°C (350°F), Gas Mark 4.

Use a vegetable peeler to create strips of the vegetables or slice them finely. Place on a baking sheet.

Toss with the oil and season well. Bake for 10–15 minutes in an even layer, turning once during cooking, until crisp and golden. Allow to cool completely on the baking sheet. Once cool, these will keep in an airtight container for up to 1 week.

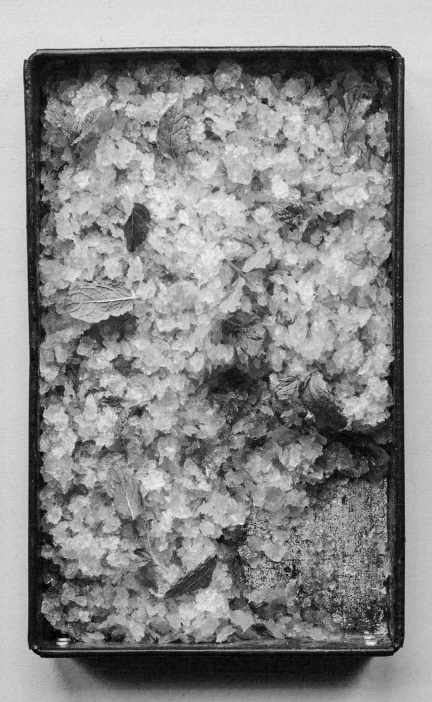

SOMETHING SWEET

MELON & MINT GRANITA

An easy yet impressive dessert of incredibly refreshing little ice crystals that melt in the mouth. Use any flavoured liquid you like: lemon, apple or mango juice, or the leftover liquid from poached fruit. You can also blend any other fruit, such as canteloupe melon or strawberries, to a purée, then pass it through a sieve and use that as your flavoured base. Any spare melon juice can be kept in a bottle in the refrigerator for up to 4 days. (See photo on page 122.)

SERVES 4-6

1 small watermelon (about 500 g/1 lb), peeled and deseeded
80 g (3¼ oz) caster sugar
80 ml (3½ fl oz) water
2 mint sprigs, plus extra to serve
3 tablespoons lime juice, or to taste

Blitz the melon in a food processor until smooth. Pass the purée through a sieve, discarding any fibres that won't pass through.

In a small saucepan, heat the sugar and measured water with the mint sprigs and stir until the sugar is dissolved, then boil for exactly 3 minutes (if you have a sugar thermometer, the syrup should reach 105°C / 221°F). Discard the mint sprigs.

Mix 500 ml (17 fl oz) of the melon purée with the sugar syrup and season to taste with lime juice, remembering that the flavours should be strong because – when frozen – they will be muted.

Pour the mixture into a shallow freezerproof and airtight container or tray and leave to cool to room temperature, then freeze for 2–3 hours. After 1 hour, stir and scrape the granita with a fork to agitate the ice crystals forming. Do this every 30 minutes for a further 1–2 hours (the time it takes will depend on your freezer).

You should be left with a crunchy, slushy mixture that should be served straight from the freezer with mint sprigs. You can also blitz the mixture in a food processor for a smoother 'slushy snow' texture.

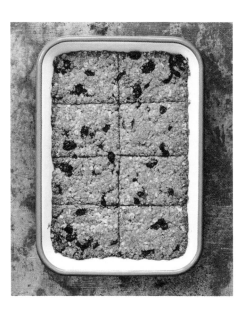

FABULOUS FLAPJACKS

Customize these flapjacks with whatever you want – try adding any dried nuts and fruit you like, or even chocolate chips.

MAKES 6 LARGE FLAPJACKS

175 g (6 oz) vegan margarine, plus extra for greasing
80 g (3¼ oz) golden syrup
250 g (8 oz) rolled oats
100 g (3½ oz) light brown sugar
75 g (3 oz) raisins (optional)
pinch of salt

Preheat the oven to 160°C (325°F), Gas Mark 3. Grease a 25 x 20 cm (10 x 8 inch) baking tin with margarine.

In a small saucepan, melt together the margarine and golden syrup.

Put the oats, sugar and raisins, if using, in a large bowl. Pour in the melted margarine and syrup, stir well to combine and add the pinch of salt.

Push the oat mixture into the prepared tin, using your hands to press it down evenly. Score the flapjack into 6 rectangles to help you to cut it after it's baked.

Bake for 25–30 minutes until golden. Allow to cool in the tin for at least 1 hour, then slice and store in an airtight container for up to 4 days.

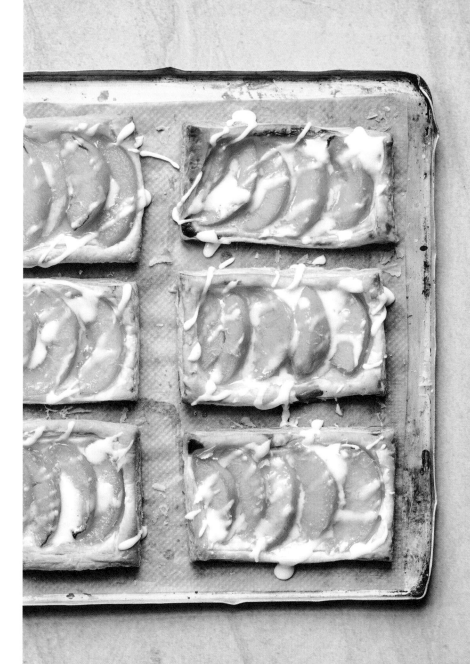

CANNED FRUIT TARTLETS

Having a stash of canned fruit and some vegan puff pastry in the refrigerator or freezer means you can whip up an economical, fuss-free pudding in no time. Swap the peaches here for apricots or mango, if you prefer.

MAKES 6

320 g (11 oz) ready-rolled sheet vegan puff pastry
plain flour, for dusting
400 g (13 oz) can peach slices, syrup drained and reserved
finely grated zest and juice of 1 lemon
100 g (3½ oz) icing sugar

Preheat the oven to 180°C (350°F), Gas Mark 4.

Roll out the pastry a little more on a lightly floured work top, trying to keep it in a rectangular shape. Cut the pastry into six evenly-sized rectangles and place on a large baking tray.

Arrange 4–5 peach slices on each pastry rectangle in a fan pattern, then brush with some of the syrup from the can and sprinkle with lemon zest.

Bake for 12–15 minutes until the pastry is puffed and golden brown.

Meanwhile, gradually add the juice of the lemon to the icing sugar until you have a thin icing of a pourable consistency.

Once cooked, allow the pastries to cool on the tray for 10 minutes before transferring to a wire rack. Drizzle each tartlet with icing and allow to set before serving.

PEANUT BUTTER MILLIONAIRE'S SHORTBREAD

This take on the classic slice is rich, on a budget. If you can't stretch to sea salt flakes, then just add a pinch of regular salt to the peanut butter filling instead, or coarsely grind some cheaper rock salt and sprinkle it on top in place of the sea salt flakes. This is best served from the refrigerator, where it will stay perfectly fudgy for up to 5 days.

MAKES 9 PORTIONS

'Shortbread'
50 g (2 oz) rolled oats
50 g (2 oz) ground almonds
2 tablespoons golden syrup
   or maple syrup
20 g (¾ oz) vegan margarine

Topping
20 g (¾ oz) unsalted peanuts
50 g (2 oz) coconut oil,
   melted
2 tablespoons golden syrup
   or maple syrup
175 g (6 oz) smooth peanut
   butter
100 g (3½ oz) 70% cocoa
   vegan dark chocolate
sea salt flakes (optional,
   see recipe introduction)

Line a 20 x 20 cm (8 x 8 inch) cake tin with nonstick baking paper in 2 strips, overlapping in a '+' shape.

Put the oats in a dry frying pan and place over a medium-high heat. Cook, stirring constantly, until they turn a shade darker and smell toasted. Tip into a bowl. Repeat with the ground almonds, then tip them into the bowl with the oats. Finally, toast the unsalted peanuts for the topping in the same way, then roughly chop them.

To make the 'shortbread', melt together the syrup and margarine in a small saucepan. Add the toasted oats and ground almonds and stir well to combine. Press this mixture evenly into the prepared tin and refrigerate while you complete the next stage.

For the topping, whisk together the melted coconut oil, syrup and peanut butter. Pour over the prepared base and allow to set in the refrigerator for 1 hour.

Melt the chocolate in a microwave in 30 second bursts or in a heatproof bowl over a pan of just-boiled water (don't let the bowl touch the water).

Pour the chocolate over the peanut butter layer, smoothing out with the back of a spoon to get it into all the corners. Top with the chopped toasted peanuts and a sprinkle of sea salt flakes, if using.

Refrigerate until the chocolate has set, then cut into 9 squares with a sharp knife. Store in the refrigerator.

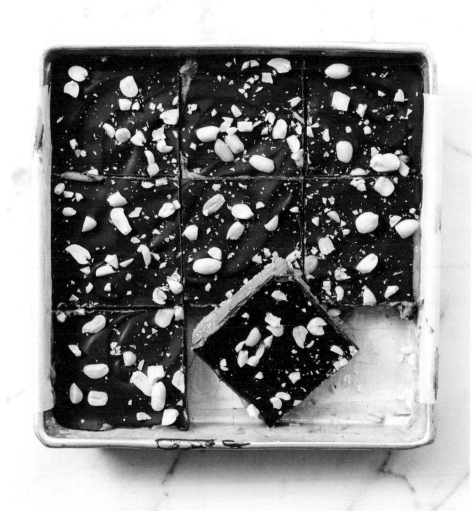

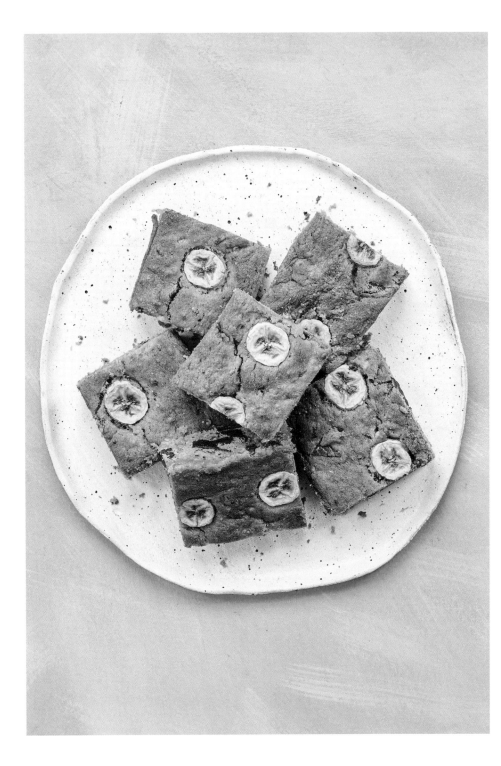

BANANA BLONDIES

These thick, fudgy bars with a taste of caramel are a great way to use up over-ripe bananas...in fact, the blacker the better. If you can get your hands on vegan white chocolate, it works really well with the blondie vibe, but dark chocolate is just as tasty. If you don't have any self-raising flour, you can just use plain flour – they will be just as delicious, they just won't rise.

MAKES 12

200 g (7 oz) vegan margarine, plus extra for greasing

125 g (4 oz) caster sugar

125 g (4 oz) dark brown sugar

3 ripe bananas, mashed with a fork, plus 1 firm banana (optional)

150 g (5 oz) smooth peanut butter

125 ml (4 fl oz) dairy-free milk

1 teaspoon apple cider vinegar

250 g (8 oz) self-raising flour

100 g (3½ oz) chocolate, roughly chopped (see recipe introduction)

Preheat the oven to 180°C (350°F), Gas Mark 4. Grease a 30 x 20 cm (12 x 8 inch) cake tin.

Cream the margarine and both sugars together until paler and fluffy, using an electric whisk. Beat in the mashed bananas and peanut butter.

In a separate jug, combine the milk and vinegar, then add half to the mashed banana mixture, followed by half the flour and mix well until fully combined. Repeat with the remaining wet and dry ingredients, then scrape into the prepared tin.

Peel and slice the firm banana, if using, and arrange on top of the batter.

Bake for 30 minutes until golden on top and risen. A skewer inserted into the centre should only have a few moist crumbs sticking to it.

Allow to cool in the tin for 20 minutes before transferring to a wire rack to cool completely. Slice into 12 square blondies.

Store in an airtight container for up to 4 days.

APPLE CAKE

This is the perfect way to use up any wrinkly apples, but it also works wonderfully with pears or rhubarb. Coating the fruit in the flour mixture makes sure it doesn't all sink to the bottom. The spices, fruit and nuts are optional – use whatever dried fruit and nuts you have.

SERVES 8

vegan margarine, for greasing

350 g (11½ oz) self-raising flour

½ teaspoon bicarbonate of soda

½ teaspoon fine sea salt

1 teaspoon ground cinnamon (optional)

3–4 apples (total weight about 350 g / 11½ oz), peeled, cored and chopped into 1–1.5 cm (½–¾ inch) chunks, plus extra (optional) for topping

75 g (3 oz) sultanas or raisins (optional)

50 g (2 oz) nuts, chopped (optional)

finely grated zest and juice of ½ lemon

75 ml (3 fl oz) flavourless oil

225 ml (7½ fl oz) dairy-free milk

2 tablespoons demerara sugar (optional)

Preheat the oven to 160°C (325°F), Gas Mark 3. Grease a 20 cm (8 inch) loose-bottomed cake tin and line the base with nonstick baking paper.

In a large bowl, combine the flour, bicarbonate of soda, salt and cinnamon, if using. Toss in the apple chunks, sultanas or raisins and nuts, if using, and coat them all thoroughly in the flour mixture.

In a smaller separate bowl, mix together the lemon zest and juice, oil and milk. Slowly add the wet ingredients to the dry and fold them in using a large spoon or spatula until fully combined.

Spoon the batter into the prepared tin, smoothing out the top. You can use one-quarter of an apple, very thinly sliced, laid out in a spiral shape on top of your cake, if you like. Sprinkle the demerara sugar over the top, if using, and bake for 1¼ hours until a skewer inserted into the centre comes out clean.

Allow to cool for 15 minutes in the tin before removing the sides of the loose-bottomed tin and popping the cake on to a wire rack. This is delicious served slightly warm, or will keep in an airtight container for up to 6 days.

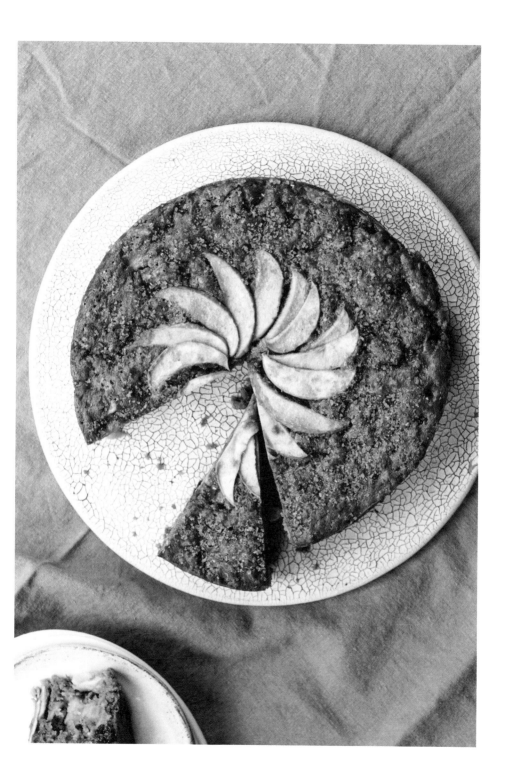

CHOCOLATE CHIP COOKIES

These have everything: rich pools of melted chocolate, crispy edges and chewy centres. The recipe halves really well, so you can make a small batch of delicious cookies whenever the mood strikes.

MAKES 8 LARGE COOKIES

150 g (5 oz) soft light brown sugar

2 tablespoons cornflour

75 g (3 oz) coconut oil, melted

50 ml (2 fl oz) dairy-free milk

1 teaspoon vanilla extract (optional)

¼ teaspoon bicarbonate of soda

¼ teaspoon baking powder

½ teaspoon fine sea salt

200 g (7 oz) plain flour

125 g (4 oz) 70% cocoa vegan dark chocolate, roughly chopped

Preheat the oven to 180°C (350°F), Gas Mark 4. Line a baking tray with nonstick baking paper.

In a large bowl, whisk together the light brown sugar, cornflour and coconut oil until just combined. Add the milk and vanilla extract, if using, and whisk for 1 minute until noticeably thickened.

Sprinkle over the raising agents, salt and plain flour and whisk again to combine. Add the chocolate and use your hand to fully incorporate it.

Using 2 tablespoons, divide the dough into 8 portions on the prepared tray. Don't worry about trying to get them perfectly round; the melted coconut oil will mean they're too soft to shape yet.

Refrigerate for 15 minutes, then roll each portion between your hands to get a uniform ball. Try to leave some of the larger chunks of chocolate on top of the cookie, to get those signature gooey pools. Leave 4 cookies in the refrigerator on a baking paper-lined plate.

Bake the other 4 cookies for 10 minutes on the tray, leaving plenty of room between each one as they will spread.

Leave to cool on the tray for 2 minutes before transferring to a wire rack to cool fully, while you bake the remaining cookies in the same way.

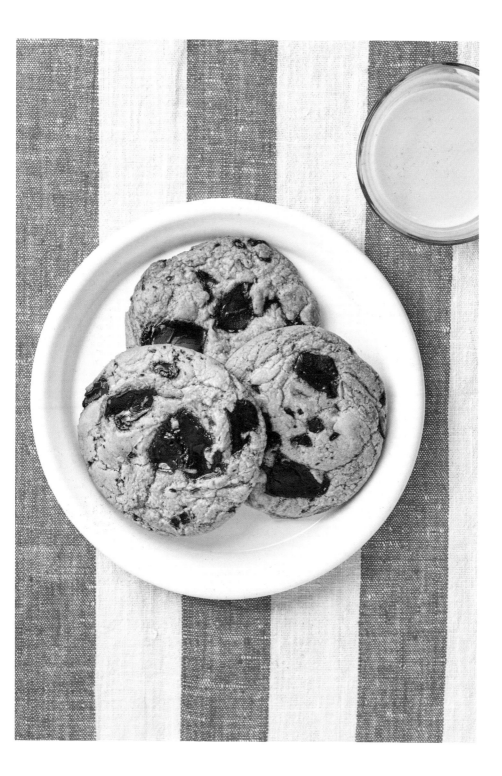

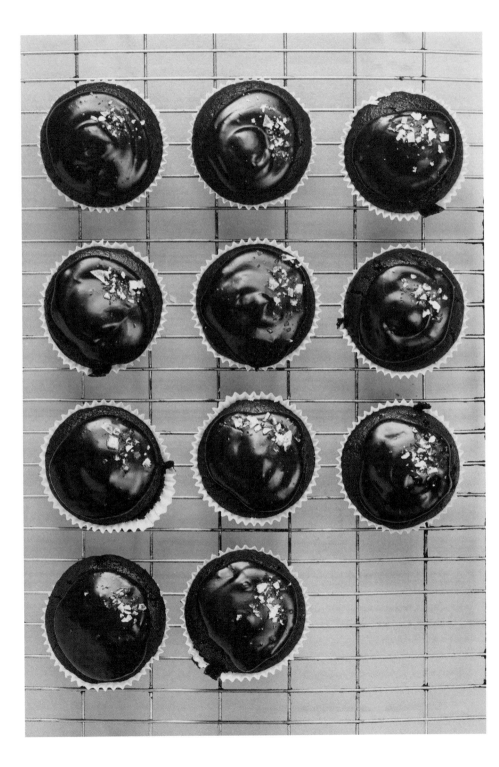

CHOCOLATE SEA SALT CUPCAKES

These cupcakes are incredibly light and rich and are highly addictive! If you don't have sea salt flakes, just add a pinch of regular salt to the chocolate icing. The coffee in the recipe brings out the chocolate flavour, but if you're not a coffee drinker just use hot water instead.

MAKES 12 SMALL CUPCAKES

Cupcakes
100 g (3½ oz) self-raising flour
100 g (3½ oz) light brown sugar
25 g (1 oz) cocoa powder
pinch of salt
75 ml (3 fl oz) hot coffee or boiling water
60 ml (2½ fl oz) dairy-free milk
60 ml (2½ fl oz) flavourless oil
1 teaspoon vanilla extract (optional)

Icing (optional)
50 g (2 oz) 70% cocoa vegan dark chocolate
50 g (2 oz) icing sugar
2 tablespoons dairy-free milk
sea salt flakes, to sprinkle (optional, see recipe introduction)

Preheat the oven to 180°C (350°F), Gas Mark 4. Line a 12-hole cupcake tin or bun tin with small cake cases, or just use squares of nonstick baking paper.

In a large bowl, whisk together the flour, sugar, cocoa powder and salt until no lumps remain.

Add the coffee or boiling water, milk, oil and vanilla extract, if using, and whisk well until you have a smooth batter.

Spoon 1–2 tablespoons of batter into each of the cake cases and bake for 14–16 minutes until firm and springy to the touch and a skewer inserted into the centre comes out clean.

Remove the cakes from the tin and leave to cool on a wire rack.

Once cool, if you are making the icing, melt the chocolate in a microwave in 30 second bursts or in a heatproof bowl over a pan of just-boiled water (don't let the bowl touch the water). Whisk the melted chocolate with the icing sugar and milk until you have a thick but spreadable icing. Top each cake with 1 teaspoon of icing and a pinch of sea salt flakes, if using.

Store in an airtight container for up to 4 days.

CHOCOLATE MOUSSE

These have only 4 ingredients! Whisking up the liquid from a can of chickpeas gives you airy, fluffy, light puddings that only take 10 minutes to whip up, and the recipe is waste-free because you can use the chickpeas for Chickpea Tabbouleh or Crispy Chickpeas (see pages 80 and 121).

MAKES 4–6, DEPENDING ON RAMEKIN SIZE

225 g (7½ oz) 70% cocoa vegan dark chocolate, plus extra to serve (optional)
150 ml (¼ pint) chickpea liquid (aquafaba)
150 g (5 oz) caster sugar
½ teaspoon salt

Melt the chocolate in a microwave in 30 second bursts or in a heatproof bowl over a pan of just-boiled water (don't let the bowl touch the water). Set aside to cool, but don't allow it to set.

Drain a can of chickpeas and measure the liquid – the amount you get varies from brand to brand, so measure it out and then use the same amount of sugar.

Put the chickpea liquid and sugar in a bowl and, using a hand whisk or stand mixer, begin to whisk. After 5 minutes, add the salt. It should take 10–12 minutes to get the mixture to form stiff peaks.

Carefully fold in the cooled, melted chocolate using a large metal spoon, if you have one. Divide the mixture between 4–6 ramekins or glasses, or put the whole lot in a big bowl and get people to dig in.

Grate chocolate on top, if you like, and allow to set at room temperature for at least 2 hours.

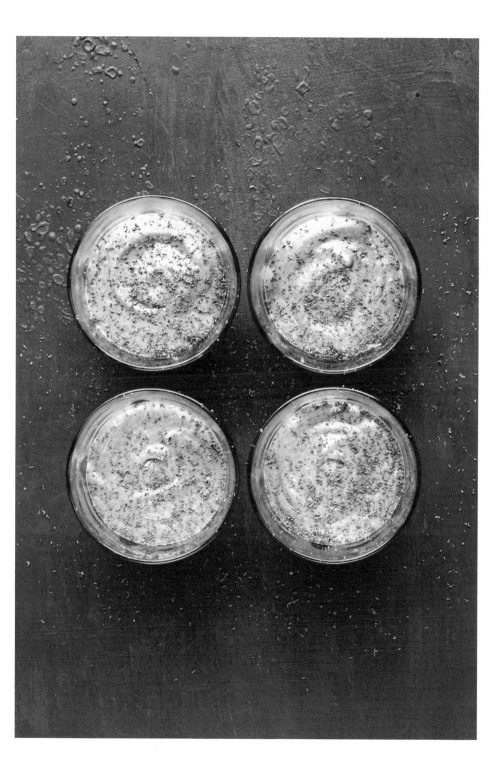

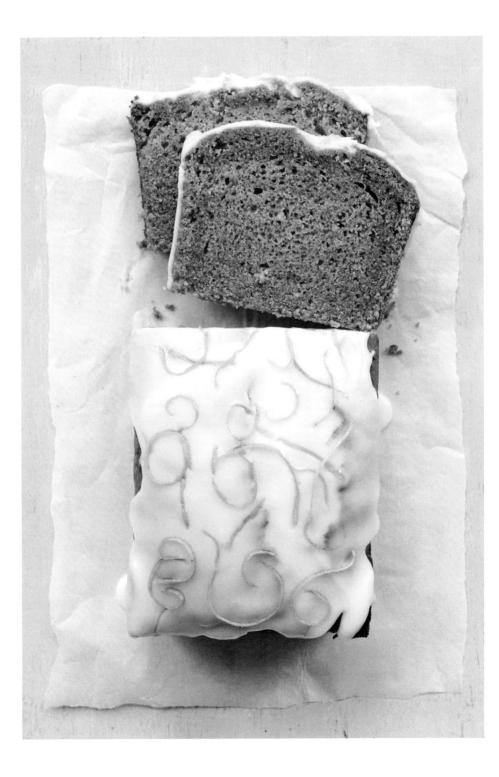

EARL GREY LEMON DRIZZLE LOAF

There's no cheaper way to add buckets of flavour to a cake than to use a few tea bags that you have lying around. Earl Grey and lemon work wonderfully together, and this loaf is so moist that it will keep in an airtight container for up to 7 days.

MAKES 1 LOAF

Cake
vegan margarine, for
    greasing
250 ml (8 fl oz) almond milk
    or other dairy-free milk
3 Earl Grey tea bags
110 ml (3¾ fl oz) flavourless
    oil
finely grated zest and juice
    of 2 lemons
300 g (10 oz) self-raising
    flour
225 g (7½ oz) caster sugar
pinch of salt

Icing
long strips of zest and juice
    of 1 lemon
100 g (3½ oz) icing sugar

Preheat the oven to 160°C (325°F), Gas Mark 3. Grease a 900 g (2 lb) loaf tin and use 2 strips of nonstick baking paper overlapping in a '+' shape to line the tin, which will help you to lift the loaf out when it's finished baking.

Put the almond milk and tea bags in a small saucepan and warm gently – you don't want to bring it to the boil, it should just be warm to the touch. Turn off the heat and stir well, pressing the tea bags against the side of the pan to infuse the milk with as much flavour as you can until it is a deep brown colour; this should take around 5 minutes. Discard the tea bags, making sure you squeeze all of the milk out of them first.

Add the oil, lemon zest and juice to the milk.

In a large bowl, whisk together the flour and sugar and salt, then slowly whisk in the wet ingredients, stirring well until you have a smooth batter.

Transfer the batter to the loaf tin. Bake for 50–55 minutes until a skewer inserted into the centre comes out clean. Leave to cool in the tin for 15 minutes before lifting out the loaf and transferring to a wire rack to cool fully.

To make the icing, slowly add the lemon juice to the icing sugar until you have a thick but spreadable icing – you may not need all the juice, because if your drizzle is too thin it will run off the loaf completely. Ice the top of the cake and top with long strips of lemon zest.

INDEX

INDEX

UK/US
GLOSSARY

UK	US	UK	US
Aubergine	Eggplant	Pulses	Legumes (dried beans)
Baking paper	Parchment paper	Rocket	Arugula
Beetroot	Beet	Salad leaves	Salad greens
Bicarbonate of soda	Baking soda	Self-raising flour	Use all-purpose flour, adding 2 teaspoons per 1 cup flour
Bouillon cube/powder	Stock cube/powder		
Brine	Salt-based liquid or solution		
		Shortcrust pastry	Flaky pastry (piecrust)
Broad beans	Fava beans	Skewer	For testing baked goods, use a toothpick
Butter beans	Lima beans		
Caster sugar	Superfine sugar	Spring greens	Collard greens
Cavolo nero	Tuscan kale (black kale)	Spring onion	Scallion
		Sultanas	Golden raisins
Chestnut mushroom	Cremini mushroom	Sweetcorn, canned	Corn kernels
Clingfilm	Plastic wrap	Tea towel	Dish towel
Coriander	Cilantro (but if the coriander seed, whole or ground)	Tomato passata	Tomato puree/tomato sauce
Cornflour	Cornstarch	Tomato purée	Tomato paste
Courgette	Zucchini	Vegetable crisps	Vegetables chips
Desiccated coconut	Unsweetened dried coconut	Wholemeal flour	Whole-wheat flour
Double cream	Heavy cream		
Fast-action dried yeast	Active dry yeast		
Filo pastry	Phyllo pastry		
Flaked almonds	Slivered or sliced almonds		
Flapjack	Oat bars		
Golden syrup	Light corn syrup		
Ground almonds	Almond meal		
Hob	Stove		
Icing sugar	Confectioners' sugar		
Kitchen paper	Paper towels		
Pak choi	Bok choy		
Pastry case	Pastry shell/crust		
Plain flour	All-purpose flour		
Porridge	Oatmeal		
Porridge oats	Rolled oats		
Potatoes, King Edward or Maris Piper	Use Yukon Gold or russet potatoes